EQUINE HOOF CARE

EQUINE HOOF CARE

Jerry Trapani

Illustrations by Rita Trapani

ARCO PUBLISHING, INC.
NEW YORK

Published by Arco Publishing, Inc.
215 Park Avenue South, New York, N.Y. 10003

Copyright © 1983 by Jerry Trapani

Illustrations by Rita Trapani
All photographs, except as noted, are by Jerry and Rita Trapani.

Library of Congress Cataloging in Publication Data

Trapani, Jerry.
  Equine hoof care.

  Includes index.
  1. Hoofs. 2. Horseshoeing. I. Title.
SF907.T7 1983   636.1'0833   82-18405
ISBN 0-668-05376-3

Printed in the United States of America

10 9 8 7 6 5 4 3 2 1

Contents

Acknowledgments

I want to thank the many clients who over the years have become friends. Without them this book could not have been written, because they shared their knowledge and experience with me.

I also want to express my thanks to Mrs. Anne Gribbons, for contributing the foreword; to Gail and Budd Benner of G. and B. Farrier Supply, for their help and the use of their shop to take photographs; to Irene Baebler and Jean and Doug Kruger, for typing my manuscript and getting a crash course in horse shoeing and horse vocabulary; and to Tony Cordero, who spent some long cold winter days photographing.

How could I even begin to thank my wife Rita who did the marvelous illustrations and put up with me. The illustrations were the easy part.

Preface

The purpose of this book is to show the importance of hoof care for the riding horse. Unlike in the past, when horses were mainly used for work, they now play a more diversified role in our leisure activities. English and Western shows, Thoroughbred and harness racing, steeplechasing, eventing, dressage, and pleasure riding—these have all turned the old workhorse of the past into the sporting horse of today.

Our equine charges and their health, therefore, are a great responsibility. The horse's main support is its hooves, and we owe it to this fine animal to gain as much knowledge of this unique structure as possible. Without proper hoof care and a thorough understanding of how the hoof works and its relation to the rest of the horse, the horse owner is somewhat handicapped in his ability to maintain the optimum health of his four-legged friend and companion.

In this book we will discuss the history and necessity of shoeing horses, accompanied by related stories, as well as how the hoof works, the proper balancing of it, choosing the right shoe for the work to be performed, various ways of correcting problems of the hoof, and how to properly trim the hoof and keep it pliable and healthy so our horses may serve us long and well. This is not meant to be a technical manual, but rather a book to give the horse owner and trainer guidelines as to proper care of the horse's feet.

The sporting horse industry of today (which probably includes about 95 percent of horses being used) is a very lucrative one and in some areas is the sole means of support of many in the field. Other related businesses—such as horse showing, saddlery and tack repair, feed and hay farms—depend heavily on the sporting horse industry. Many charitable organizations raise a good bit of their money by running horse shows and horse-related activities. Pony clubs and 4H clubs teach school-age children to become knowledgeable, productive, and happy adults.

The racing industry, as you can see by some of the headlines in newspapers, is a billion-dollar industry in itself. With the prices that stallion shares and mares are now bringing at sales, especially in New York with the New York State Breeders Program, sizable awards are made to encourage New York-bred horses to be raised and run in this state. As a result, many new people are being attracted to the horse industry. Therefore, I think there is a great need for a book such as this to help fill in the gaps and make the horse owner more understanding of the whole animal.

There is an old European saying: "No hoof, no horse." Nothing is more true than this statement. Without the hoof, the horse cannot perform any job properly. Even horses that are used only for breeding purposes must be sound enough to be turned out to pasture, and broodmares must carry the added weight of pregnancy. Therefore, trimming the feet and keeping them well balanced and healthy is of primary importance. Without proper shoeing and hoof care, the performance horse cannot do his job.

As the book progresses, you will see that horses need various types of shoes to perform these jobs. Racehorses require special shoes to grip the track and give them the necessary traction to come out of the starting gate and gain as much ground as possible with every stride, while the jumper must be able to jump safely, land, and make sharp turns without slipping or falling and causing injury to himself or his rider. A trail horse used on endurance rides must have special shoes so that he can travel a hundred miles without wearing them out or having to stop for long rest periods. Proper shoeing and hoof care keep a horse in condition and lengthen his years of service.

If you have ever purchased new shoes which were uncomfortable for the first few days or hours, you may remember that they gradually shaped themselves to your feet, becoming more comfortable. Horseshoes do not have this ability. They are made of steel or aluminum, and it is the farrier's job to trim the hoof and fit the shoe without error. If it doesn't fit right the first time, it will be uncomfortable for the horse, sometimes causing chronic lameness. When we come home at night, we can kick off our shoes, put up our feet, and relax. Unfortunately, our horses can't do this. A farrier's job is very important, because the shoes must fit properly.

I believe there is a need for some sort of nationwide farrier certification, not exactly a licensing, program that would list farriers and their backgrounds, so that a horse owner could find a farrier, look at his certification, find out whether he is an apprentice, journeyman, or master farrier, and determine his suitability. As a farrier, I feel that it is only fair that experienced farriers be given proper recognition for their years of work and study.

Foreword

Anyone involved with horses in sports or in competition knows the truth of the saying, "No foot—no horse." All the best supplements, training, and showmanship will do you no good at all if the horse is not sound. The actual meaning of "soundness" is relative to the game you play, and in my field (which is dressage), it means more than just being able to get around. Small irregularities in a horse's gaits are of vital importance in the dressage arena when purity of movement is at a premium.

It was a pleasure to meet and get to know Jerry Trapani as a farrier because he showed interest in and understanding of more than just "getting the tires on." Jerry would come and watch the horse travel over the ground before he started shoeing him. He would take time to discuss a problem without becoming impatient with "owner-interference" and, most of all, he could usually fix the problem. Jerry Trapani has trimmed and shod our breeding stock and farm horses for years now, as well as my show horses.

In addition to being pleased with his work, I value Jerry's steady temperament around the animals and his realistic attitude toward his trade. If Jerry makes a mistake, he'll admit it and correct it instead of covering up and getting defensive. And I have yet to hear him belittle a colleague or scream in horror when viewing the work of another farrier: *Who* shod this horse?!! He is confident and plain-spoken, just like the book you are about to read.

I especially enjoyed the chapters on balance and the common lameness problems because the suggestions for correcting the problems are stated briefly and are right to the point. For experienced horsemen, there will be little revealed in this manual which they don't already know—and yet a review as easily digested as this one can be most beneficial. The novice around horses will find a multitude of clear, no-frills advice he can make repeated use of in the future. As a reference to return to, Jerry Trapani's book will earn its place in your library.

ANNE GRIBBONS

EQUINE
HOOF CARE

1

Why Horses Need Shoes

The horse, as used today for pleasure or sport, needs shoes to protect its feet from wear.

In the old days, horses were run down a dry riverbed by wranglers until their feet became sore, whereupon they were easily captured and broken. Once the feet grew out, they were shod and ridden again.

While practices have changed, the horse has not. A horse ridden without shoes for a long period of time over a hard surface will wear its feet down until they are sore. When the human fingernail is torn below the skin line, it is very sensitive. We do not have to walk around on our fingertips, but the horse, in a sense, does, and he therefore needs protection.

Shoeing is a "necessary evil" for the jobs that we have given our horses to do. It should be done in a natural manner so as not to encumber or detrimentally affect the horse's natural way of going. Shoes can also be used to correct various conformation and gait defects that cause the horse to interfere, stumble, or become lame. Corrective shoeing and balancing are wonderful therapeutic tools. If used properly, they can keep an older horse or a horse with some problems serviceably sound for a number of years.

Horseshoes are basically made of two materials: steel and aluminum. Aluminum shoes are used for specific purposes. Because aluminum is softer and lighter than steel, it is more easily

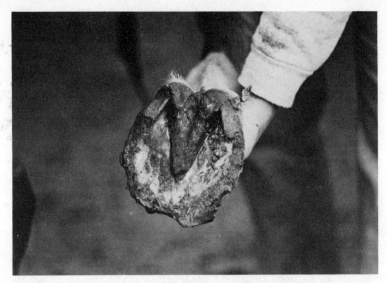

Hoof badly in need of farrier care. Note broken walls.

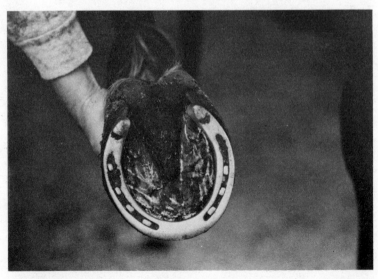

Here, the hoof wall has overgrown the shoe at the heels; this could cause corns and cracking of the heels.

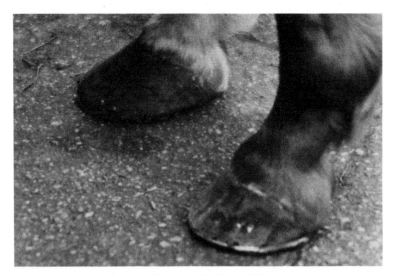

One foot properly trimmed and shod. Note difference in hoof angle.

shaped but wears out more quickly on the horse's foot. The softness of aluminum allows the horse some added comfort over a steel shoe and the lightness in weight allows you to use a wider shoe, thus covering more of the horse's foot for protection, as opposed to steel. Steel shoes last longer and are used on most horses. Aluminum shoes are used only on show horses and racehorses, who go on fairly good surfaces, either on racetracks or in riding rings. The advantage of an aluminum shoe on a show horse is that its lightness does not encumber the horse, allowing it to show all its natural movement. Sometimes, however, a horse needs a slight bit of weight on its shoes to encourage it to use itself better, especially in the case of saddle horses, where heavy steel shoes are used with toe weights to encourage the horse to give us that high-stepping gait so well known to the breed.

While on the subject of weight on horseshoes, imagine your horse's front leg as a pendulum swinging from the shoulder. The average horse's front leg is about three feet long. Each ounce of weight on the end of that pendulum at its highest point of swing

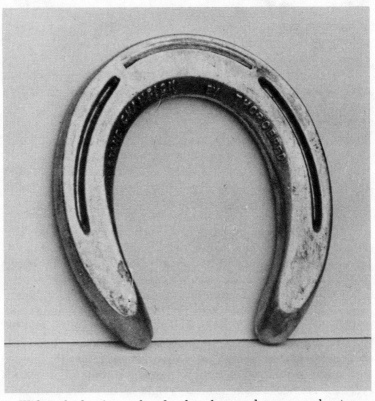

Wide-web aluminum shoe for show horses, dressage, or hunter.

is increased by twenty-two times its weight. Therefore, a ten-ounce horseshoe has the downward force of 220 ounces pulling down on that horse's leg. Imagine picking up a water bucket with your arm. If it is empty, you can lift it up straight away from your body, but if that bucket were full of water, you would have to bend your elbow first and then move it away from your body. This same principle explains why heavier shoes usually give a horse more knee action. A lighter shoe will allow a horse to move in a low sweeping stride that is popular in some divisions, such as hunters and dressage. Weight placed at the toe of the foot will encourage the horse to follow that weight and take a longer stride. Some Standardbred horses, especially trotters, will have lead or brass toe weights screwed onto the wall of the foot to encourage them to take a longer stride and, therefore, cover more ground. Side-weighted shoes will have a similar effect, whereby the foot will follow the weight. In other words, if a side-weighted shoe has the weight positioned on the outside branch of the foot, the foot will swing outward to allow the horse more clearance. This shoe is used sometimes on pacers (also Standardbreds) who, because of their lateral gait, have a tendency to cross-fire and knock themselves rather badly. This is a fairly severe correction and should not be used on every horse.

Corrective shoeing should be done in stages, starting with the least effective and seeing what works best. Sometimes it takes many shoeings to find the correct combination for each horse. If a horse does have a problem, corrective shoeing can sometimes make an improvement so that the horse may later be returned to more normal shoeing, or, at least, to a milder correction.

The foot must always be trimmed level so that it strikes the ground evenly on both sides, or branches, as they are called. If you watch a horse walk away from you directly from the back, both heels of the foot should strike the ground at the same time, not one before the other. If you watch the horse from the side, the foot should come down as close to level as it possibly can. In most cases, the heel will strike the ground a split second sooner than the toe; then the horse will roll over the toe, causing the normal wear pattern on the shoe, which is equal all around and slightly more worn in the center of the toe. If a horse's shoes show that he is stabbing his toes into the ground and wearing out his shoes much faster than he should, the foot is probably out of balance or

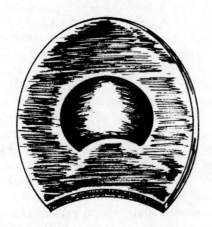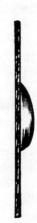

Anti-snowball pad.

the horse's heels are hurting him. Consequently, he wants to put his weight on his toes first and then rock back over the heel.

The frog is the shock absorber of the foot. As the frog strikes the ground it spreads the heels and distributes the concussion of hitting the ground evenly up the leg. That is why the heel lands slightly sooner than the toe. The frog works in partnership with a balanced foot. An out-of-balance foot landing sideways could literally shatter the bones in the foot. This condition often happens to racehorses and fractures the bones of the ankle and the sesamoid. As a horse becomes fatigued, the muscles and ligaments become tired, causing them to lose their resiliency and their ability to work properly. If a tired racehorse does not change his lead or is too tired to switch properly, he could break down in the stretch run because of this. It is not necessarily the fault of poor shoeing, but related to other factors.

For the riding horse, especially a horse who jumps over uneven ground, such as a field hunter or event horse, a foot that

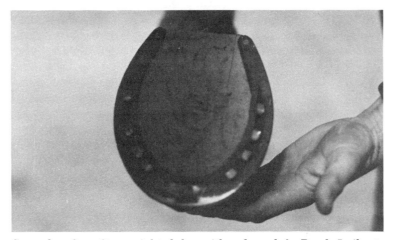

Ground surface of toe-weighted shoe with pads made by Randy Luikart at the AFA Convention, 1982.

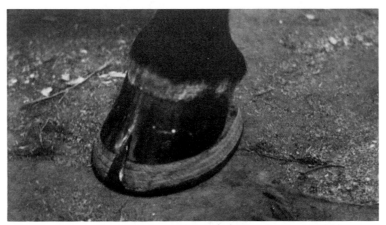

Toe-weighted shoe with pads and welded clip by Randy Luikart, 1982.

is out of balance can cause a myriad of problems further up on the leg, in ankles, splints, knees, and right on up through the shoulder. Each bone in the whole leg column is related to the

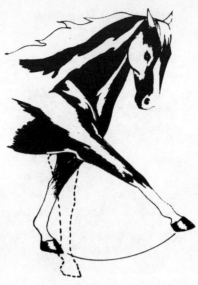

The pendulum effect. The weight of a shoe on the hoof at the leg's fullest extension is multiplied approximately twenty-two times. For a low, sweeping stride, light shoes are used, while a high-stepping, knee-snapping action is achieved by the use of heavier shoes.

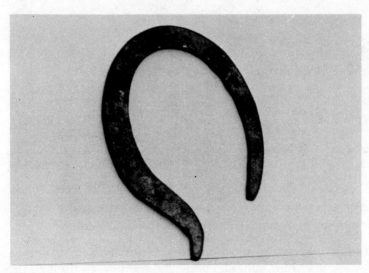

Side-weighted shoe with trailer.

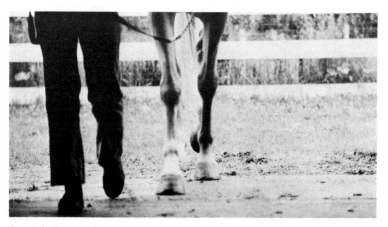

Straight legs and balanced feet. Note proper placement of all four feet.

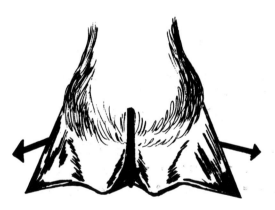

Direction of frog pressure. As the hoof strikes the ground, the frog spreads downward to the ground surface, allowing the heels to spread outward, relieving pressure on the sensitive structures above. The common belief of lowering the heels to increase frog pressure is not a good practice, because examination of the feet of wild or unshod horses will show normal expansion despite the apparent lack of frog pressure from long heels. Domestic horses, however, should have their feet trimmed and balanced for sanitary reasons.

other and everything must fit together in proper alignment for the horse to be sound and remain sound. Some horses have conformational defects, such as sprung knees or a foot that is not placed directly underneath the pastern bone. These are fairly common problems and can be dealt with through proper trimming and shoeing of the horse.

TRACTION

Shoes must sometimes be applied for traction to enable the horse to grip and move off the ground with greater ease. Racehorse shoes have a high steel toe grab and heels (or what are called stickers) on the hind shoes. Good traction is necessary going out of the starting gate, having the horse settle into a long stride, and for easy gaining of ground. At the racetrack, you will sometimes see flashing lights on the tote board next to a horse's number or on a separate equipment information board that indicate the type of shoes that the horse has on. Shoes that afford good traction can affect a horse's performance tremendously, especially on "muddy" or "sloppy" tracks. Many trainers will have their racehorses reshod, if it has rained the morning of a race, with special shoes called mud calks. Mud calks give the horse even more traction than normal shoes. There are also special shoes for use on turf courses; they are designed not to pack up with the turf, which can be very slippery if wet.

Riding horses also need a certain amount of traction. For the average pleasure horse, flat shoes with a small crease called a fuller will give enough traction for normal riding. Sometimes a small heel is applied to the hind shoes to add a little more traction. Horses that are doing more strenuous work—for example, jumpers or event horses that must go over varying terrain—are sometimes fitted with special removable calks. These calks are screwed into holes that are drilled and tapped into the shoes, thus eliminating the need for removing the shoes and renailing them back on to change the traction requirements. Sometimes different-sized calks will be interchanged during events. Imagine having to get your horse shod between each class because it rained or the footing in front of a single

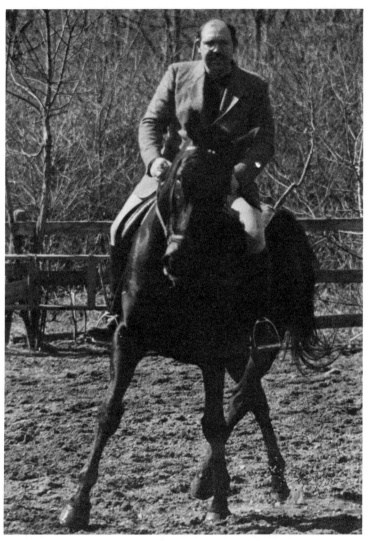

Jerry Trapani riding St. Elmo's Fire (Thoroughbred). Calks give horses confidence to move forward boldly in adverse conditions, such as slippery turf, ice and snow, and muddy ground. *(Photograph by Terri Miller)*

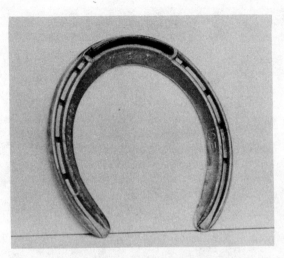

Front aluminum racing plate with steel toe grab.

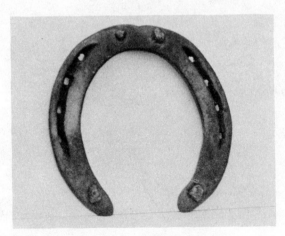

Wide-web front shoe with fuller and borium, good for field hunters or eventing horses.

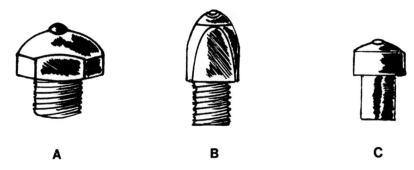

A   **B**   **C**

Three types of calks. *Figure A* is a small, screw-in type suitable for field or show hunters and dressage horses. *Figure B* is larger and sharper and also removable. This is suitable for eventing horses and jumpers. *Figure C* is a drive-in calk, is not removable, and provides suitable traction for horses of any discipline.

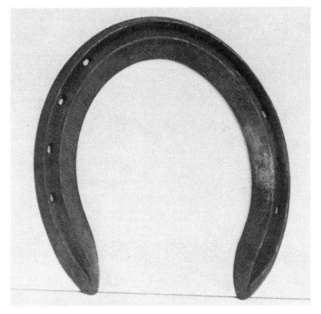

Steel training plate for young horses or racehorses.

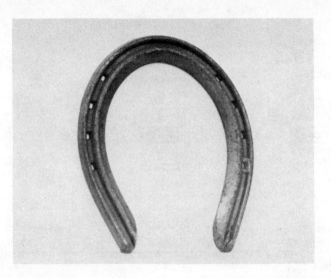

Rim shoe. Note that it is heavier than a training plate and suitable for showing or field work.

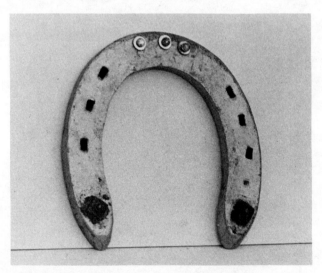

Aluminum shoe with screw-in calks and steel wear tabs.

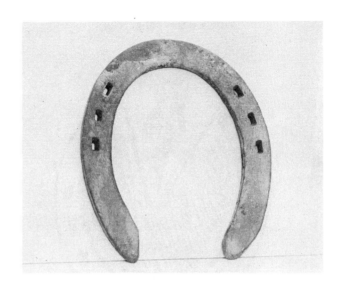

Quarter-by-¾ front shoe.

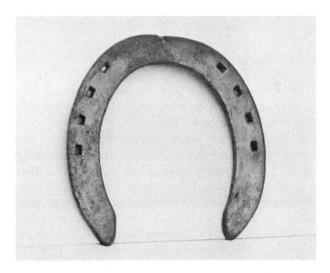

Handmade ¼-by-⅞ front shoe used for light horses.

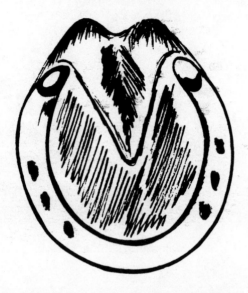

The placement of the nail holes in the shoe should correspond to the outer border of the white line and not be placed any further back than the widest part of the hoof.

jump has gotten sloppy! This would ruin the horse's feet and hold up the whole show!

There are also calks that are nonremovable. These are called drive-in calks. A hole is drilled, the calk is applied, then peened over the underside. These are usually smaller than the screw-in type but still allow very good traction. The carbide alloy borium is sometimes welded to shoes in different patterns to give the horse traction and allow the shoes to last longer. Borium is a very hard surfacing material and comes in different-size grit. Usually a spot is put at each heel, as well as at the toe of the shoe. The borium digs into the ground surface, giving the horse traction. Horses that are driven or ridden on roads, such as police horses, have a smoother type of borium applied, especially at the toes, to give the shoes a longer wearing period.

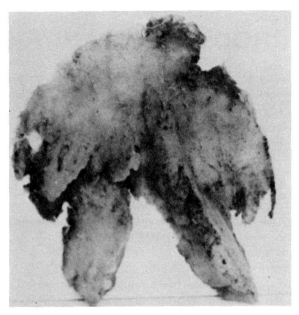

Silicone packing showing impression of frog and sole.

There are also various types of shoes that affect traction. I mentioned a fullered shoe earlier. This shoe has a small rim in the area of the nail hole. This rim fills with dirt, and the friction of the dirt against the ground surface gives a slight bit of traction. A swedge or rim shoe has the rim totally surrounding the shoe. This fills with more dirt, consequently giving more traction. Aluminum shoes afford a little more traction than steel shoes; the wear on the shoes is greater and faster, since aluminum is softer. The indentations thus occurring in the aluminum cause small ridges that add sometimes to traction, especially on grass. However, the width of the aluminum shoes on show horses sometimes negates this. For riding in winter conditions on snow or ice, there are nails called ice nails which have hardened tips that protrude above the surface on the horseshoe. These tips will dig into the ice and afford the horse traction.

CHOOSING THE SHOE

A normal shoeing job should be done with the horse's use in mind. On most horses, flat shoes or small heels on the hind feet will do nicely. The web of the shoe, or the width, should be approximately ⅓ more than the width of the wall outside the white line. On the average, a shoe should be approximately ⅝ to ¾ inches wide. In cases of broad, wide feet, a width of ¾ to ⅞ of an inch should be used to distribute the weight better over the bearing portion of the foot and not put too much weight on the wall, as this will cause cracks and breaks. The nails should be placed no further back than the bend of the wall toward the heel. In other words, the last heel nail should not be placed beyond the widest part of the hoof.

Pads on the horse's feet should be limited to use only for protection, or if the horse has a problem due to conformation or illness. If a horse had a broad, flat-footed sole with not much concavity to it, pads are a good means of protecting the sole from bruising.

In a normal foot, the sole is concave, allowing for movement up and down and protecting the coffin bone lying inside. On a flat-footed horse or a horse that has had laminitis, the sole is closer to the ground and is thinner. Consequently, it will bruise more easily, so a pad made of plastic or leather should be applied. The packing under the pad can consist of various materials; pine tar and okum are the normal packing materials. In some cases, you can use foam rubber or silicone. There are also acrylic preparations that are similar to silicone in that they do not dry hard, but remain soft and absorb more concussion. I believe that pads should not be left on a horse constantly unless there is a physical need for them. The pads take away from the normal action of the foot, and the frog has a tendency to trap dirt and moisture, causing thrush. If your horse does require pads, you will not be able to clean under them. Flushing this area periodically with a thrush preparation is advisable to help kill any bacteria before it can cause problems.

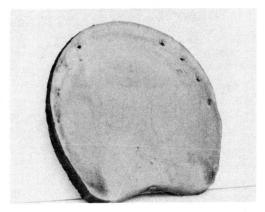

"Three-degree" pad used to elevate the heel to relieve soreness.

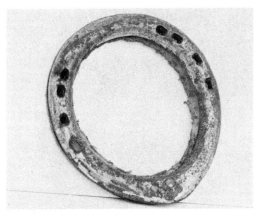

Half-round egg-bar with rim pad.

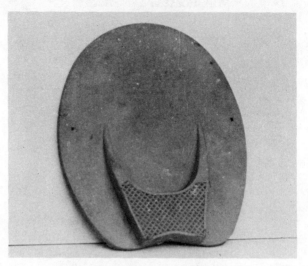

Heel cushion pad. This is suitable for contracted heels, navicular disease, or for protection of the frog area if required.

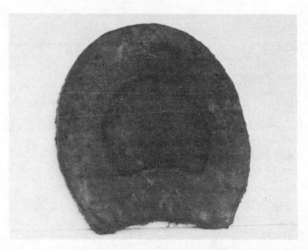

Anti-snowball pad. Use of this pad prevents snow from balling up in the horse's hoof.

LAMENESS

At times, due to conformation or lameness, we must change the angle of the hoof by using shim pads or degree pads. They come in various thicknesses ranging from two degrees to four degrees. Occasionally, on some three- and five-gaited horses, the pads are applied in many layers to increase the length of foot and change the angle for a flashier stride. If a horse just requires padding directly under the shoe, e.g., on a flat-footed horse, you may not want to cover his sole completely. You may raise the hoof surface off the ground with rim pads. The rim pad is cut to the exact size of the shoe itself and riveted with a copper rivet at the heel to prevent it from shifting while under the horse.

Applying a wider-webbed shoe to distribute the weight better and give more support will help a horse that is sore-footed without having to apply pads. When pads are taken off, special care should be taken that the foot does not become dry and brittle, because a dry, unpliable foot will bruise more easily than one that is healthy and pliable. A good hoof preparation used a couple of times a week will help prevent this problem.

Venus of Turpentine is another good material which will help toughen the feet, keep them healthy, and encourage growth. It is most effective when heated to a semi-liquid form, then painted on the soles. This will give the soles resiliency and help prevent bruising. Needless to say, the horse's use and the terrain over which it is ridden are the deciding factors as to whether or not the feet need to be toughened or pads are required. Each horse is an individual, and the health of its feet must be taken into consideration accordingly.

Bar shoes can also be used to prevent lameness or take pressure away from a certain area of the foot. In cases of quarter cracks, a bar shoe should be used to take pressure off the affected area, allowing the crack to heal itself and grow down from the coronary band. Enough room should be left under the crack to slip a hacksaw blade underneath, so that no pressure will be applied to the crack. The bar takes the weight off the frog and keeps the foot stable. As soon as the crack is healed, the bar shoe

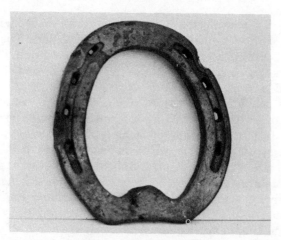

Bar shoe with three clips to stabilize hoof crack.

should be removed to encourage full use of the foot again.

A horse which has had laminitis or founder should be shod with a very wide-webbed shoe, and the bearing surface should be concave to keep the pressure off the flat convex sole. Sometimes a rim pad is applied, and in more severe cases, a full metal or aluminum pad is applied over the plastic one. A horse which is foundered can still remain sound and useful through proper shoeing. The foundered horse will want to put more weight on his heels. If the feet are left unattended, the toe will sometimes curl completely up off the ground, giving that "Aladdin's slipper" effect that we sometimes see in feet left unattended for long periods of time. This is a very bad situation and should not be allowed to happen.

Sometimes separations will occur at the hoof wall, either at the quarter or at the toe. If this happens at the toe, we call it a "seedy toe." This is usually from improper trimming. The foot is not trimmed level, and foreign material such as sand or dirt gets wedged under the shoe and works itself deeply into the laminae or white line. If this happens at the quarters, we call this condition a "gravel," and this gravel may occasionally work its way right up through the wall, breaking out at the coronary band. This is very painful for the horse, requiring that the pressure be removed and the foot soaked. Once the pressure is relieved, the hoof should be closed up with a wide-webbed shoe and a pad. Silicone should be applied underneath during the time the foot is allowed to grow out. Careful trimming of the foot is necessary.

If your horse is lame shortly after being shod, there may be several reasons. Sometimes the sole is not pared away properly, and it will rest on the shoe. If the shoe comes in contact with the sole, it will create pressure, causing the horse pain. Sometimes nails are improperly driven, not necessarily into the quick, but just close enough to bulge the laminae out to the sensitive portion. If this be the case, once the nail is removed, the horse should be sound in a day or two. If the farrier has quicked your horse and blood is apparent, the nail should be removed and the hole flushed out with peroxide. If the horse has not had a tetanus shot recently, he should be given one. Soaking the foot for a day or two is a good idea to remove any dry blood and prevent infection.

If the sole is pared down too far and begins to bleed, the use of a pad or rim pad to take the pressure off that area is indicated until the foot can grow out to its normal proportions again.

The outer wall of the hoof should not be rasped indiscriminately. There is an outer covering called the periople that grows down from the coronary band. This is the natural coating of the hoof that helps keep the moisture in. Rasping should be done only from the area of the nails down. Hoof dressing should be applied directly to the hoof again after the farrier is finished. In some cases, if there is excessive flaring of the hoof, the farrier must rasp away this flaring to help balance the foot again. Hoof dressing should then be applied immediately after shoeing and special care taken to see that the hoof does not dry out. Hoof dressing should not be applied too often, because some dressings have a tendency to cake up on the hoof. This may rot the wall underneath, causing what is called "punky feet." Nails holding the shoe will be unable to take a good hold, causing loose and lost

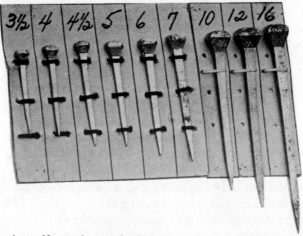

Various sizes of horseshoe nails. Smaller nails are used on ponies and racehorses, medium-size nails are used on light horses, and larger nails are used on gaited horses, enabling the farrier to nail through many layers of pads.

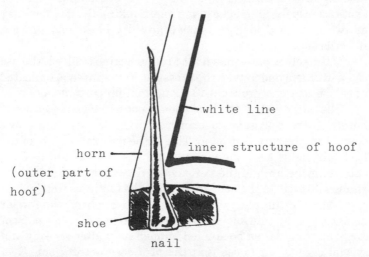

Nail placement is extremely important. The nails should be driven approximately ⅝ of an inch high and in an even line. If they are driven too high, they can place pressure on the sensitive structures or quick the horse, and if placed too low, they will not hold properly and will split the hoof wall.

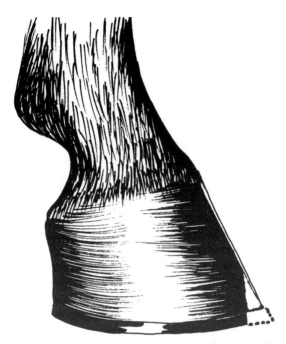

Dumping of the toe. The shoe should be fitted properly to the contours of the hoof wall. When the shoe is allowed to slide back or is not fitted properly in the first place, the unsightly and improper practice of the dumping of the toe occurs. The dotted line indicates where the shoe should have been fitted.

shoes and further damage to the hoof.

The size and amount of nails are very important. A good rule of thumb is never to use a nail any larger than is required. Usually six to eight nails are the maximum. Six good nails will hold a shoe as well as eight, so if your farrier can use six, your horse is better off. The nails should be placed outside the white line and come out approximately ⅝ of an inch high, then clenched down with a small clench to keep them from pulling out. If the use of clips is indicated on your horse because of broken feet, they should not be too large and should never be applied too close to the white line.

2

History of Horseshoeing

THE HORSESHOER

When we hear the term "marshal," many of us picture a law officer. The word is derived from several Frankish and Norman words which translate as "horse-servant." Marshals were placed in charge of the care of cavalry horses in early times. Marshals came from England to France and, as in many occupations, those performing the job of marshal took that word as their surname. The seventh Earl of the English Earls of Pembroke, Walter Marshall, used a horseshoe and nails on his seal in the 1200's. Even though the duties of marshal were later changed somewhat, the marshal set the stage for professional horse care as we know it today. Among these special duties was that of farrier.

The blacksmith's prestige rose with the advent of the iron horseshoe. His services were more essential, as he now performed the job of shoeing war horses and chariot horses in addition to making armor, weapons, and tools. As tribes and nations expanded their territories via conquests, the increase in the blacksmith's duties made it necessary to specialize, thereby producing armorers, blacksmiths, and farriers. The word "farrier" itself is derived from the Latin term *faber fariaris,* which means to work or fabricate with iron.

The blacksmith came into being with the discovery of iron as a workable metal as far back as 2,500 to 3,000 years ago. The Hittites of Asia Minor were the first to begin to work iron on a large commercial scale, using it as a means of trade and barter with their neighbors. It was through this trading that iron reached Europe. The Greeks were the next to utilize this metal, and in the fifth century B.C., iron and its many uses became known in Britain.

Ordinary men must have been quite impressed with the first blacksmiths, who could wield and shape inflexible material by means of heating it in fire. Blacksmiths themselves were well aware of their power and were careful to keep the secrets of working iron items, and their longevity (as noted in the many iron artifacts we have today) made the good blacksmith a much sought-after craftsman.

The actual shoeing of horses did not occur until some 400 years later, when around the ninth century, man began to create artificial roads. Prior to this, animal shoes were not essential. The Greek hippo sandal, a primitive shoe, seemed more like a hobble than a protective device when strapped to the foot of the horse. The iron horseshoe we know today was not used then either in Greece or by the Roman cavalry in Britain, even though the cavalry was greatly utilized at the end of the Roman era. In those days, riders would wisely dismount and lead their horses over difficult terrain. Tough-footed mules served as mounts to save the more delicate feet of the horses on hard, uneven ground. We have evidence that metal plates were tied to damaged feet as protective devices. Man took this a step further, subsequently fitting shoes to healthy feet to prevent injury.

History reveals that Celtic and Germanic tribes shod their horses with iron plates and nails even before the Roman conquest. These tribes were quick to assimilate useful items such as iron, as the knowledge of it aided in their own survival and gain. It is difficult to think that the farriers we take for granted today held almost magical powers in the eyes of ninth-century man. The Druids also may have been familiar with the art of working iron and may have, among their duties, served as blacksmiths to

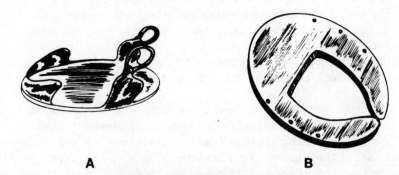

Figure A. Roman hippo sandal of
the first century A.D. *Figure B*.
North African horseshoe of the
twelfth century.

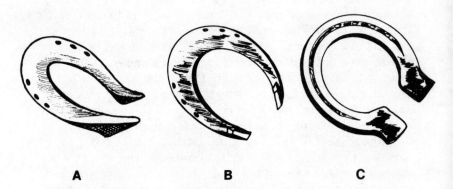

German horseshoes. *Figure A*. Thirteenth century. *Figure B*.
Crusades. *Figure C*. Fifteenth century.

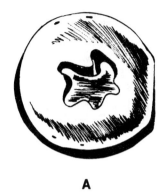
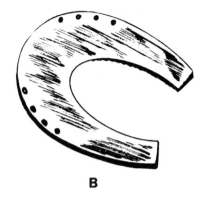

A **B**

Spanish horseshoes. *Figure A*. Twelfth century. *Figure B*. Nineteenth century.

shoe horses for battle. A highly secretive people, the Druids hid their art well from the Romans, whose history does not mention horseshoes and accompanying equipment until the ninth century A.D.

Blacksmiths and farriers had their own patron saints in several countries. Often, the patron saint was a skilled craftsman in the art of metalworking and was greatly revered by those in the trade.

France's St. Éloi, born in A.D. 588, was an artisan's son schooled in the art of metalworking, specifically gold. A very religious man, Éloi founded a monastery and a nunnery in France upon land given him as a gift for his dedication and excellent craftsmanship. His ability for making thrones and other complex metal items distinguished him as a craftsman.

In several old engravings of St. Éloi, we notice that he is often pictured holding the leg of a horse. There is a story that a horse, claimed to be possessed by the Devil, was brought to him for shoes. Éloi promptly cut off the leg of the undisciplined, prancing animal, shod the hoof, and miraculously replaced the leg without a scar on the horse's body. This sensational act brought Éloi more fame than his expert craftsmanship in metal. St. Éloi also served as Bishop of Noyon for nineteen years.

St. Dunstan of England is honored as that country's patron saint of blacksmiths. St. Dunstan was born of a West Saxon noble family related to the ruling family at that time. As a youth, Dunstan served at King Athelstan's court, but was cast out due to a disagreement. Upon the suggestion of his uncle, the Bishop of Winchester, Dunstan then took up the monastic life. He returned to his home near Glastonbury and withdrew to a small cell to pursue a life of prayer and manual labor. Also skilled in metalwork, Dunstan fashioned church vessels and bells of fine quality.

It seems these devoted blacksmiths had more than their share of visitations by the Devil, and St. Dunstan was no exception. Legend has it that one evening, while quietly working at his forge, Dunstan was visited by the Devil disguised as a beautiful woman. Not to be fooled, Dunstan grasped the woman quickly by the nose with a pair of red-hot tongs. The Devil's resulting howl was so great that the force of it cracked the cell's rock foundation into three sections.

The same story has different endings in different parts of the country. One version has the Devil leaping wildly and landing with such force that a flowing spring erupted from the cracked ground. In another, the Devil, disguised as a horse, seeks Dunstan out and asks to be shod. Dunstan deliberately causes the Devil great agony in shoeing him and stops only when he has made the Devil promise never to enter any structure upon which a horseshoe is hung. This is the reason we see so many horseshoes hanging above doors.

Travelers on horseback honor St. Martin of Tours as their patron saint. St. Martin's emblem contains a horseshoe, and many travelers often hung a horseshoe in their homes to ensure a safe return.

THE HORSESHOE

Domestication of the horse took place around 3000 B.C., with his use as a riding and work animal commencing around 1600 B.C.

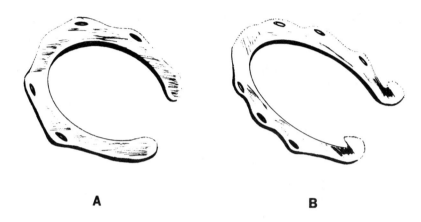

A   B

Figure A. Sixteenth-century Hunish horseshoe. *Figure B.* Chinese horseshoe of the early twentieth century.

This increased use necessitated the protection of his feet, as first recognized by the Egyptians and Persians. Woven-reed shoes attached to the feet in a sandal-like manner prevailed in China until the 1800's and may still be in use today. Leather moccasin-like footwear for horses was also used as a means of protection.

Much of twelfth-century Genghis Khan's military success was due to his development of a rawhide covering which fit closely and securely around the hoof. This allowed for more mobility and protection for the horse. As the horse's use increased, so did the importance of the blacksmithing trade. Specialization in the creation of farriers' supplies became more evident, as the art of horseshoeing was a time-consuming operation. Since the 1200's, both horseshoes and nails were available as ready-made items to European horseshoers. The black-smithing trade in general was highly respected, as it continued to be the foundation of most industry.

In early America before the mid-eighteenth century, the shoeing of horses and oxen was relatively rare, due to the high cost of importing iron from Europe. During the nineteenth century, several machines for the production of both horseshoes and horseshoe nails had been invented and perfected. America's westward migration saw many groups traveling, each with its own blacksmith, upon whose craft they depended for equipment repair and the shoeing of horses and oxen.

Today there are many large companies producing quality farrier tools and supplies. Good materials are in great demand to properly equip the sporting, pleasure, or competition horse, as well as for the rebirth of the horse's use as a work animal. Farriers still fashion handmade shoes, but good machine-made shoes have lightened their work burden, allowing them to concentrate on the primary concern of correctly balancing and preparing the horse's feet.

FIGHTING INFLATION

With today's spiraling inflation, the costs of all our necessities are skyrocketing. Prices rise drastically on everything we buy, with gasoline, fuel, oil, feed, hay, and bedding at or near the top of our lists. The price fluctuation of these items, especially for the horse owner who cannot buy and/or store them in large quantities, can be depressing.

There is one facet of your "horsehold" that has held the line against inflation: the shoeing of your horse. Fifteen years ago, when I began working, the going price in my area for a basic shoeing job was fifteen dollars. Today, the average price is around twenty-eight dollars. That is only a bit more than 70 percent increase over fifteen years. Consider our dollar's worth then and now. A good horseshoer makes a decent living for a

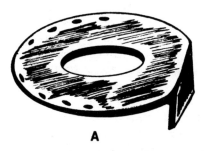 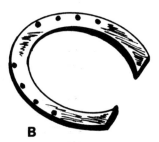

A   B

Figure A. Fourteenth-century English horseshoe. *Figure B*. French horseshoe from the Crusades.

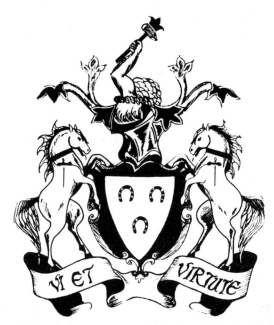

Crest of the Worshipful Company of Farriers, seventeenth century. The Worshipful Company of Farriers was a guild organization dedicated to ensuring high-quality workmanship among horseshoers, and its origins have been traced back as far as the 1300's.

long, hard day's work, but his cost of living has risen right along with everyone else's.

Here is a breakdown of the rise in costs of the basic materials and equipment needed by your farrier: Steel has risen 500 percent in the last fifteen years, with 300 percent of that increase having taken place within the last five years. Horseshoes, horseshoe nails, and components of the farrier's own tools are made of steel. Truck prices have risen 250 percent. In 1965, a new pickup truck (no frills) cost about $2,500. Today that price hovers around the $8,000 mark. We all know what the cost of gasoline has done to us in the last five years! And those little extras, such as pads, silicone, and borium, have increased substantially in price. A number of these products are petroleum-based, such as some of the special types of shoes and pads.

It is doubtful that these figures will trigger a panic among horse people, or that farriers around the country will raise their prices en masse. Farriery is an art and a labor of love. If it weren't, there would certainly be more complaints about the decrease in our profits over the past decade and a half. If farriers raised their prices according to every wave in the economic ocean, horsemen's expenses would be greatly increased. Perhaps now you will understand why having your horses done regularly on your farrier's route is appreciated, and why your farrier might have to charge you for a special trip to replace a lost shoe the evening before a hunt or a show.

3

Anatomy and Physiology

A horseshoer needs to have a working knowledge of the anatomy and physiology of the horse's leg from the knee down. Competent mechanics don't try to overhaul engines unless they thoroughly know their parts and their functions. A horseshoer also needs to know the workings and the mechanisms he is called upon to overhaul. He is working with a living creature. Veterinarians learn anatomy and physiology before they learn surgery.

A knowledge of some basic anatomical terms is useful in the study of the anatomy of the horse's leg. These basic terms are: **hoof**, the horny covering on the end of the horse's leg and **foot**, the hoof and the structures contained within it. The terms hoof and foot are often used interchangeably. The **leg** is the portion of the limb of the horse below the knee or hock. **Digit** is the portion of the leg below the **fetlock**. **Limb** is the leg and the structures above it that join it to the trunk of the horse. **Medial** is the inside plane of any structure. **Lateral** is the outside plane away from the center of gravity of the horse.

The front limbs carry about 65 percent of the horse's weight. The center of gravity of a horse is above and about six inches behind the elbow. The front limbs have mainly a supporting function and push down when the horse moves. The hind limbs have more of a driving function. The horse pushes off them when moving. There are differences between the front and hind limbs;

35

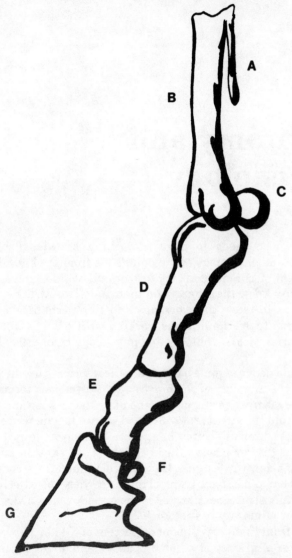

Bones of the front leg. *A*. Bottom of the splint bone. *B*. Cannon bone. *C*. The sesamoid bone. *D*. The first phalanx or long pastern. *E*. The second phalanx or short pastern. *F*. Navicular bone. *G*. The third phalanx or coffin bone.

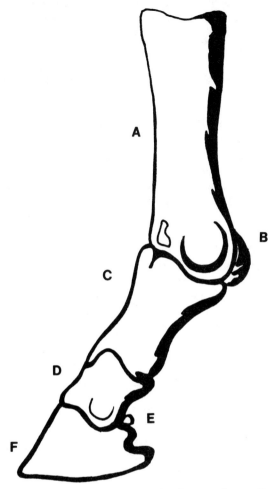

Bones of the hind leg. *A*. Cannon bone. *B*. Sesamoid bone. *C*. First phalanx or long pastern. *D*. The second phalanx or short pastern. *E*. The navicular bone. *F*. The coffin bone. Note that the long and short pastern bones are steeper than those of the front leg and are somewhat shorter.

the upper portion of the front and hind limbs have entirely different structures from the knee end of the cannon bone up, but are essentially the same from that point down to the coffin bone. The common names for the bones below the knee and hock joint are the same for both front and hind legs. Other less obvious differences between the front and hind legs are that the hind leg has a longer and thicker cannon bone and a more upright pastern bone. The hind leg also has a more oval hoof and a more concave sole.

All the bones of the leg have cartilage at their ends to allow for bone growth. The growth pattern of the leg can be affected by the distribution of weight on the cartilage. Corrective trimming is some help up to the time that this line closes, usually when the horse reaches two years of age. Radical changes can be made in the legs of very young foals by a process called stapling. The maturity of race and performance horses can be determined by radiographs of this line. All bones of the legs have an articular cartilage on the joint surfaces. These cartilages are extremely smooth and slippery and allow great freedom of movement. They also bear weight. They fuse when a condition called "dry joint" takes place. This is known as ankylosis or fusing of the joint.

The cannon bone is located just below the knee and has the bones of the knee bearing upon it. The front cannon bone is oval shaped and flat on its front surface. The hind cannon bone is thicker and longer than the front one, somewhat rounder in shape and slightly pointed in front. The function of the cannon bone is to support and bear weight. It is subjected to a terrific amount of stress. No manmade structure of similar proportion could withstand the force placed on it at speed. The cannon bone also functions as a lever. The relationship between the length of the cannon and the length of the pastern bones has been shown to affect the speed of horses. A relatively short cannon bone in relation to a long pastern seems to be the most desirable combination in terms of creating leverage for speed and reducing concussion to the upper legs.

The symptoms of shin buck or shin splints are the result of irritated or torn periosteum on the front of the cannon bone. This is due to poor conditioning, coupled with overexertion. It is very common in young racehorses first put in training.

The splint bones are located on either side and in back of the cannon bone. Their upper ends form part of the bearing surface of the knee. When a foal is born, the splint bones are not attached to the cannon bone by bone, but by ligaments. The splint bones usually fuse naturally to the cannon bone by the time the horse reaches the age of six. The splint bones are shaped like long-drawn-out triangles and have small nodules on the pointed ends. The function of the splint bones is to protect the tendons and ligaments, and especially the blood vessels and nerves, which pass down the back of the leg and provide greater bearing surface for weight by supporting a portion of the knee joint. The inside splint bone usually bears more weight than the outside. The inside splint bone supports a portion or two of the knee bones, while the outside bone only supports a portion of one. An inside bone can be easily distinguished because it has two facets or bearing surfaces, and an outside bone has but one. The increased stress on the inside bone is a contributing factor to the appearance of splints; thus they are more common on the inside of the leg. Splints are hard bumps formed by a tearing of the bone skin between the splint bone and the cannon bone. The irritation of the periosteum caused by the movement of the splint bone against the cannon bone from the sprain or rupture of the ligament causes calcium deposits in the damaged area. If the irritation remains, the bony growth continues to enlarge until irritation ceases or the calcium immobilizes the irritation.

The sesamoid bones are located at the back of the fetlock joint next to the cannon bone. The sesamoids are shaped like small pyramids. They are held in place by many ligaments. Occasionally one of the ligaments may become torn. This is known as a popped sesamoid. An inflammation of these bones is called sesamoiditis. Sometimes these small bones fracture as a result of a heavy blow or a severe strain. The function of the sesamoid bones is to act as a fulcrum for the ligaments and tendons which support and move the leg. The sesamoids also create a larger surface for rotation of the fetlock joint and thereby strengthen the position of the cannon bone in the joint.

The long pastern bone is located between the fetlock joint and the pastern bone. It is shaped somewhat like the cannon bone, but is much shorter, usually about one-third the length of the cannon bone on an ideally proportioned horse. The function of the pastern bone is to increase the flexibility of the fetlock joint and thereby reduce concussion. The length, flexibility, and angle or slope of the pasterns strongly influence the smoothness of the horse's gait. The angle and the flexibility of the shoulder and arm also determine the smoothness of the gait. A few degrees' difference in angle may make a difference in the desirability of the gait. Horses with relatively long pasterns and short cannons are the most desirable as speed horses because of the possibility of increased leverage. However, very long and very sloping pasterns are a weakness, causing the probability of bowed tendons and other unsoundness.

The short pastern bone is located between the long pastern and the coffin bone and is one of the bones which makes up the coffin joint of the foot. Approximately one-third of the short pastern is encased within the hoof. The short pastern bone is nearly cube-shaped. Its ends are rounded in a manner that allows the foot to twist or move from side to side in order to adjust to uneven ground.

Calcium located on either the short or long pastern bone and not involving the joint is called false ringbone. It is usually caused by a severe blow to the area. The navicular bone is located between and underneath the short pastern bone and the coffin bone; it is part of the coffin joint. The navicular bone is somewhat boat-shaped and comparatively very thin. The navicular bone acts as a fulcrum for the deep flexor tendon, which passes directly under it and attaches to the semilunar crest of the coffin bone. The location of the navicular bone makes it very susceptible to injury. Not only is it compressed by the pastern against the taut, deep flexor tendon during movement, but it is easily bruised and occasionally punctured because of its position over the center of the bottom of the hoof. The coffin bone is completely encased within the hoof or box of horn. The ideal shape of the hoof is determined a great deal by the shape of the coffin bone. The front feet have rounded, flattened, and wide coffin bones, as a rule, and the hind feet have pointed, comparatively steep and narrow coffin bones. The shape of the last third of the hoof in the heel region is not determined by the coffin bone, since the lateral cartilage which attaches to the wings of the coffin bone extends into that area. Another function of the coffin bone is to provide a surface and structure for the attachment and protection of the blood vessels and nerves which make up the sensitive structures of the hoof and form a hydraulic cushion between the bone and the hoof. The coffin bone is extremely porous and therefore very light and fragile and subject to fracture. The coffin bone is also the point of attachment for the main tendon, which causes movement of the leg. The main extensor tendon has its main insertion in the extensor process of the coffin bone. The deep flexor tendon has its insertion in the semilunar crest of the coffin bone.

THE JOINTS

The true knee of the horse is the stifle joint. Racehorses, jumpers, and other performance horses stand a greater chance of frequent knee injuries. An injury to the knee can result in a condition called carpitis, also known as "pock knee." Carpitis has a tendency to develop into somewhat large calcium deposits in the injured area. These growths result in a condition called knee spavin.

The hock joint of the hind leg corresponds in position to the knee of the front leg of the horse. The hock is similar in structure and function to a man's ankle joint. It is located between the tibia and the cannon bone and splint bones. When injury occurs to this area and calcium is formed in the joint, a condition called bone spavin arises. Bog spavin is the term for any distension of the protective hock joint capsule. All these conditions contribute to the decreased flexibility of the horse's joints, and, therefore, alter its performing abilities, depending on the severity of the condition. Fast stopping and working may cause bog spavin (e.g., in dressage horses and reining horses) because of the increased use of the hocks.

The fetlock joint is the joint where the cannon bone and the long pastern bone meet. The cannon bone itself, the two sesamoid bones, and the long pastern bone make up the fetlock joint. Moving in two directions only, the fetlock is a perfect hinge joint. The fetlock is supported by several ligaments, bands of tough tissue connecting the bones to each other. The largest of these ligaments is known as the suspensory ligament. The horse's foot in motion is more stable due to the fetlock joint's limitations for lateral movement. Corrective trimming, however, has little direct influence when trying to correct limb deviations above the fetlock. The fetlock absorbs shock and bears weight. It is subjected to great stress at high speed. The fetlocks of racehorses nearly touch the ground when they are running, as has been shown in slow-motion photography. The stress resulting from high speed causes, at times, one or more of the ligaments to sprain. This sprain can develop into calcium deposits in the fetlock area, creating what is called an osselet. In any case, healthy, springy fetlocks are desirable in riding horses, because they make the horse's gaits very comfortable. Wind puffs or wind gall is the name for the distension of the fetlock capsule.

The pastern joint is located between the long and the short pastern bones. Like the fetlock joint, it is a hinge joint, but it is an imperfect one, as it also has a slight degree of movement laterally in addition to its two main directions. The pastern joint is not as flexible as the coffin joint, but corrective trimming will be effective in bone alignment in this joint, unlike the fetlock joint. The pastern joint absorbs shock and adjusts to uneven terrain and the twisting, changing movement of the horse's feet. The position of this joint and its movement limitations increase the possibility of joint lameness and sprains. When calcium forms in the pastern joint, it is called high ringbone.

The coffin joint is located within the hoof between the short pastern bone and the coffin bones. Included in the coffin joint structure is the navicular bone. Like the pastern joint, the coffin joint is an imperfect hinge joint, allowing considerable side-to-side or lateral movement. This joint enables the horse to stand, adjust, and move with comfort on uneven ground. The coffin joint absorbs a great deal of concussion. The position of the navicular bone makes it possible for a great deal of concussion from the short pastern bone to be transferred to it and its suspensory ligament, conducting the concussion away from the delicate coffin bone. In addition, the navicular bone acts as a fulcrum, working with the deep flexor tendon in flexing the horse's extended leg. Another absorber of concussion is the elastic plantar cushion, which is located just above the frog within the horse's foot. This cushion is compressed by the downward motion of the pasterns. The compression of the plantar cushion against the frog on the ground pushes the lateral cartilages out of the quarters of the wall, which also move slightly, further reducing concussion. When calcium forms in the coffin joint, we call it low ringbone. The navicular bone is often affected, causing what is called navicular disease, which is unfortunately common because of the location and structure of the navicular bone within the hoof. Navicular disease usually begins as a bursitis in the navicular bursa between the deep flexor tendon and the navicular bone. In its late stages, navicular disease may involve not only the navicular bone but the coffin joint as well, as do advanced cases of low ringbone.

TENDONS AND LIGAMENTS

Tendons and ligaments are made of strong cordlike bands of tissue fibers. The long tendons enable the muscles of the horse's upper leg to move the foot and the lower leg as if by remote control, since there are no functional muscles below the knee or the hock of the horse. Tendons connect muscles to bones. The function of tendons is mainly to move the body. Ligaments connect bones to bones and are generally more elastic than tendons. The main function of ligaments is to support the body and its parts. When the tendons tear or rupture, they often bow. Bowing is a condition which occurs when the superficial flexor tendon tears away from the deep flexor tendon. In severe cases, the tendon sheath and ligament attachments of the tendon sheath also rupture. The chances for a horse's recovery without resulting scar tissue are very low when the tendons are strained, stretched, or ruptured. The term "strain" is used to describe excessive stretching or rupturing of muscles and/or tendons. A "sprain" refers to a condition in which the ligaments are stretched or torn, but the bones are not dislocated. Another term for dislocation is luxation. There are small lubricating saclike cushions which are located between the two opposing surfaces of a bone and a tendon. These are called bursa, and they contain a lubricating fluid called sinovial fluid. Inflammation or injury of the bursa is called bursitis. Navicular bursitis, also known as navicular disease, is common in racehorses and in some riding horses. Sometimes a false bursitis develops in the form of a shoe boil or a capped hock. A shoe boil is a buildup of fluid at the point of the elbow caused by shoes which are too long or by large calks on the shoes. It is caused when the horse lies down and folds its front legs under itself. The resulting inflammation can be alleviated by putting a shoe-boil boot on the horse's ankle or by properly fitting the shoes with heels filled so that no sharp edges are present. Capped hocks are buildups of fluid on the point of the hock, which occur from kicking in trailers or in stalls.

Tendons are protected and lubricated by sinovial sheaths, as tendons must often travel long distances over bones, other tendons, or ligaments. The sinovial sheath is a fluid-filled sac which surrounds the tendon, and when it becomes inflamed, the resulting condition is called sinovitis. When a tendon bows, the sinovial sheath of the flexor tendon is often involved.

4

Hoof Structure

The hoof is a box that surrounds the sensitive structures of the foot. It is made of many parts, all of which must be healthy in order for the horse to function properly. The hoof, if examined under a microscope, appears close in structure to hair, dispelling the common belief that it is a horse's fingernail. This explains the smell of burning hair when a hot shoe is applied to the hoof wall.

The first parts of the hoof that we normally see are the insensitive external parts: the wall, frog, sole, and periople. The wall is the outer layer of horn, which appears to be hard and woodlike. However, in reality, it is flexible, or should be on a normal hoof, and bends around the toe into the quarters and into the heels. It is most flexible in the heel area, where it meets the bars of the hoof and forms a bridge to help strengthen and support the horse's body weight and keep the heels from tearing with every stride.

The sole also appears to be a rigid structure, but this is also false. With every stride, the sole flattens slightly and bulges outward to absorb extra shock. Its main function is to protect the sensitive tissues beneath and to soften the blow of concussion to the coffin bone resting inside. A healthy sole is covered with a protective layer of dead, flaky material. This should not be pared away, but left as an additional layer of protection against bruising and such.

The frog is the triangular-shaped elastic structure in the center of the foot between the bars and the sole. A healthy frog

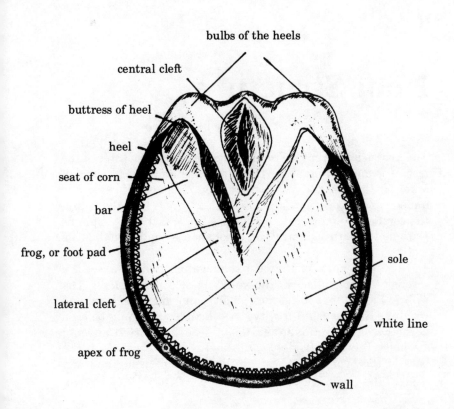

Underside (bearing surface) of a front hoof.

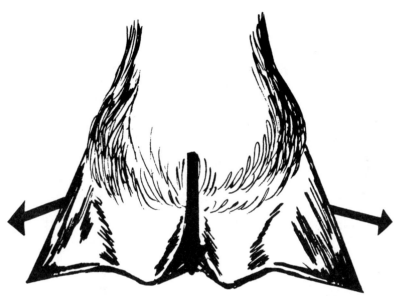

Direction of frog pressure. As the hoof strikes the ground, the frog spreads downward to the ground surface, allowing the heels to spread outward, relieving pressure on the sensitive structures above. The common belief of lowering the heels to increase frog pressure is not a good practice, because examination of the feet of wild or unshod horses will show normal expansion despite the apparent lack of frog pressure from long heels. Domestic horses, however, should have their feet trimmed and balanced for sanitary reasons.

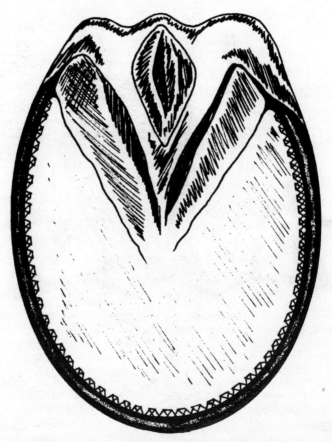

Underside (bearing surface) of a rear hoof. Note all structures remain the same, except for the actual shape of the rear hoof, which is more narrow and a bit pointed.

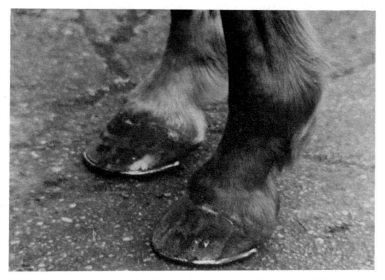

Both feet properly shod. Notice correctness of alignment with pastern.
(Photograph by Anthony Cordero)

has the consistency of a pencil eraser and has a multifaceted job to do concerning the proper function of the hoof. One of the functions is to act as a blood pump to send blood back to the arterial system of the leg. Another job is to be a cushion for the navicular bone and soft connective tissues above it. It is also a wedge that, with every stride, pushes the hoof wall and bars outward to distribute the concussion over a much larger area.

The periople is a thin layer of horn which begins at the top border of the coronet band and bridges the gap between the soft tissue and the harder hoof wall. This is very important to future growth of hoof wall, because any injury to this periople will show up in succeeding growth as abnormalities, such as cracks or deviations in wall growth. The other function of the periople is to hold moisture into the hoof by sealing the upper ends of the horn tubules in the wall.

The rate of growth of the wall seems to vary from horse to horse; on the average, however, it takes about nine to twelve months to grow from coronet band to the ground. A healthy hoof on an active horse grows faster than a dry hoof on a horse confined to a stall.

The white line, or laminae, is located beneath the wall and can be seen upon examination of the hoof from the ground surface. It is more resilient than the wall and, therefore, aids in dispersing shock through the foot. The layers of the wall and the sole come together and are held together here by a complex weaving of the laminae.

THE SENSITIVE OR INTERNAL FOOT

The coriom, or sensitive structures of the foot, are the deeper layers of skin that supply the blood and nutrition to the corresponding insensitive parts of the foot. They are: the sensitive sole, sensitive frog, sensitive laminae coronary coriom, perioplic ring, and the plantar cushion.

Starting from the top, the perioplic ring serves to give the periople its nutrition. The coronary coriom is a thick, half-round structure which lies in the coronary groove above the sensitive laminae and gives nutrition and moisture to the wall.

The sensitive laminae run in a vertical direction and are comprised of two layers forming a complex weave. They do the most to give the foot support and act like a bridge to dissipate concussion. It is interesting to note that when the galloping horse supports all his weight on one foot, the union of the sensitive laminae dovetail to give more than eight square feet of support in a capsule only about ten inches in circumference.

The sensitive sole feeds the horny sole and is attached directly to the bottom surface of the third phalanx bone.

The digital or plantar cushion is the true shock absorber and early warning system of the horse's foot. It is located in the posterior part of the foot above the frog and sensitive frog. It is a broad wedge-shaped structure whose rear portion is attached to the bulbs of the heels. It is filled with blood vessels and nerves and tells the horse over what kind of terrain he is traveling.

FOOT FUNCTION

There are two functions of the foot, to dissipate shock and to reduce slippage.

The ill effects of concussion are taken up by the complex bridgework and angulation of the bones and joints of the limbs, as well as the relatively small movement of the structure of the hoof. Even though the hoof is made of many different parts, its function must be considered as a whole. Since most of the initial concussion of stride is taken at the rear of the hoof, the most important shock absorbers are located in the rear: the frog digital cushion and the bars. Each stride of the gallop brings the entire weight of the horse onto one foot at a time, and the added weight of the mass passing over it creates a downward force of many thousands of pounds. The hoof is an engineering master-piece, where a few square inches of surface can absorb and diffuse such great pressure. Therefore, a healthy hoof must have all its factors working well in order for the horse to perform and remain sound. Almost ninety percent of all lameness occurs in the front legs, and a great portion of this is either directly caused by or brought on by improper foot care.

The anti-slippage device of the foot comes into play in the fact that the bearing surfaces of the foot, the wall, the sole, and the frog all act together to help the horse maintain his balance. The sole is concave and shaped like an inverted saucer, and when weight is placed on it, it flattens slightly, forming a tight grip to the ground surface. The frog, which is wedge-shaped with its three grooves, is the first part of the foot to come into contact with the ground. This wedge opens up and grips the surface, reducing lateral slippage, keeping the foot straight under the horse's body. The combination of the saucer of the sole and the wedge of the frog helps the horse perform properly.

A barefoot horse is better off than a shod one, but because of the work we ask, conformation problems, or bad conditions, our horses must sometimes be shod. Therefore, a thorough knowl-edge of the mechanics of the hoof must be known to the farrier and the owner alike. Here are some guidelines that should be followed when trimming a foot or shaping a shoe:

1. The wall should be trimmed to its natural proportions.
2. The outer edge of the shoe should fit fully around the outline of the wall. Excessive rasping of the wall should not be done. This could cause damage to the periople and remove the natural varnish needed on the hoof wall to prevent drying. Dumping of the wall to fit the hoof to the shoe is a gross error and should not be done or tolerated.
3. The sole should only be pared lightly to remove any flaky sole and to bring it back to its concave shape. The

sole is the protective layer between the ground and the sensitive structures above it.

4. Short shoeing, or opening of the heels, should not be done, because the bars are there to help support weight and disburse concussion.

5. The frog should also be trimmed only to remove any ragged edges and bring it back to its natural shape. A large healthy frog is important to good hoof function.

6. If a shoe is to be fitted, it must be level and of the proper size and type for the horse's job. Don't put racing plates on a trail horse or broncos (standard shoes) on a dressage horse.

7. Use as little a nail as possible and the smallest amount of them to secure the shoe properly. A #4 nail will hold as well as a #6 if placed properly and used in the correct shoe. Also, make sure there are no nails beyond the widest part of the hoof to restrict movement of the heels.

5

Balance

Throughout the book, various references will be made to the balance of the horse's foot. This balance is the alignment of all the bones, ligaments, tendons, and structures of the horse's limbs. This balance is important to the well-being of the horse because unequal pressures put on the foot are transmitted throughout the leg.

The proper trimming of the foot is achieved by observing the horse walking toward you, away from you, and from the side. The important criterion here is that you should look to see that the foot strikes the ground evenly and also leaves that way; this is called "breakover." Both heels should absorb an equal amount of weight; otherwise, a condition called "sheared heels" could occur. This is the tearing of the soft cartilage which holds the heels together. It is painful to the horse, because this area of the foot is the shock-absorbing center of the limb. When observing the horse coming toward you, the toe should breakover at the center or close to it. Observation from the side should show the foot striking the ground evenly, not heel-first or toe-first. This angle is determined by the bone structure of the leg. The pastern bones must all be in alignment for the tendons and ligaments to work properly. Front feet of Thoroughbred horses are usually 50 to 53 degrees, while cold-blooded types and European bred horses tend to be 52 to 55 degrees. The hind feet are usually steeper in angle, with 52 to 55 degrees being the most common in all horses.

Observation is the best guide, since these are not rules, but

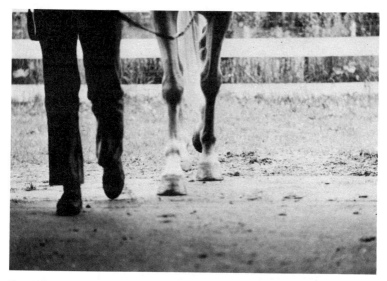

Straight legs and balanced feet. Note proper placement of all four feet.

guidelines to follow. A good way to check lateral balance of the heels is to hold the front leg up by the cannon bone and let the foot hang naturally, so that you are able to sight down directly over the frog. Imagine a T-square dissecting the frog squarely, so that both heels appear to be equal in length. Some horses, because of deviations in their limbs, need to have one heel trimmed slightly lower than the other in order to achieve proper balance. If this T-square effect is properly executed, the square should go through the foot directly up the cannon bone. Hind-foot balance is checked the same way, only you must look over the hock and check the heel.

The medial balance from the side is observed both while the horse is standing and while it is in motion. Before the farrier trims the foot, he should know where he wants to trim. This is similar to the process a sculptor goes through when looking at a rough piece of stone, making notations as to where to cut to

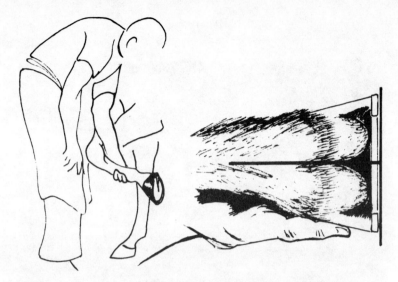

The T-square effect. An imaginary line should be drawn through the cannon bone and through the horse's heels and a T-square imagined across the ground surface of the hoof. When these factors are in alignment, this limb is balanced. Even if one heel appears slightly longer than its mate, this is nature's way of compensating for deviation. Always check the horse in motion to make sure that the hoof is striking evenly on the ground surface.

achieve his goals. Balance is the most important aspect of shoeing horses. Even if they do not wear shoes, the feet must be properly balanced. Many cases of lameness are due to improper balance, ultimately requiring corrective shoeing to restore the foot. Corrective trimming and applying the proper shoes to achieve balance is the job of the experienced farrier.

Feet that are out of balance can sometimes grow into grotesque shapes. A severely foundered foot, unattended, will grow quickly at the toe and actually curl up like an Arabian slipper. Feet that are not properly balanced laterally will grow flares outward and cause paddling or interference, and occasionally the frog may even be pushed sideways. This condition prevents the frog from performing its job as a shock absorber for the foot and encouraging circulation, and reduces the frog's elasticity.

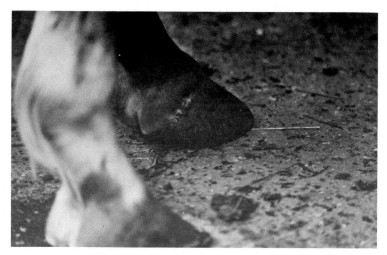

This horse's hooves have greatly overgrown the shoes. Note broken hoof axis in both feet. *(Photograph by Anthony Cordero)*

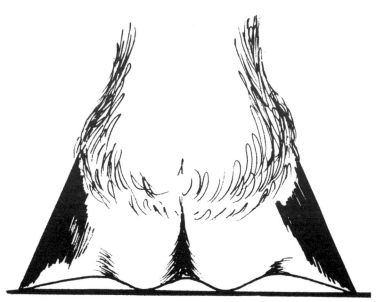

Even distribution of weight on the heels. Heels should be balanced level to distribute the weight evenly during each stride.

The foot, in general, tends to grow toward length; in other words, the shorter side will tend to stay short, while the longer side will grow faster because of less pressure, adding more problems. Horses who have limb deviations should be trimmed or shod often to keep their feet properly balanced. Many slight problems can be resolved through proper care.

6

Types of Shoes

There are almost as many types of shoes as there are horses. For every discipline of riding or sport, specific shoes are used on horses to enhance their performances, for example, in racing, jumping, dressage, eventing, and polo. Reining and endurance horses have special shoes, as they have special needs. Shoes can add or take away traction or enhance a gait, as in the case of Tennessee Walkers and Saddlebreds. They wear specially weighted shoes and shim pads to create that high-stepping action the crowds like so well. These shoes function according to the same principle applied to lifting an empty bucket. You can usually lift an empty bucket with a straight arm from your shoulder, using an almost effortless swing. This is the way a show hunter or dressage horse moves. If you fill the bucket with water, however, the added weight makes you bend your elbow first as you attempt to lift the heavy bucket. The weighted shoes and pads on Saddlebreds create this same effect, as the horses must first lift their feet up, then out. The foot tends to follow the weight. On some trotters, toe weights are screwed to the toes of their feet to make them reach for the track with each stride. Weights placed on the sides of shoes tend to make the feet swing wider and allow more clearance so the horse won't interfere.

Polo ponies make quick stops and sharp turns and accelerate very quickly, so their traction requirements are great. They wear rim shoes with a higher inside rim. The groove or swedge fills with dirt, creating an abrasive layer against the turf. The inside rim gives better traction while allowing extra clearance for those tight turns. Barrel racers wear similar shoes, but with

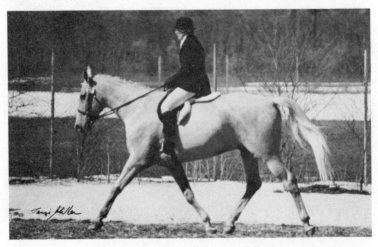

Rita Trapani riding Ganymede (TB Cross). Note the low, sweeping stride of the show hunter ("daisy cutter"). *(Photograph by Terri Miller)*

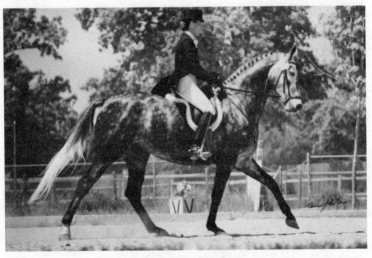

Anne Gribbons riding Kristall (Swedish Warmblood), USDF First Level Horse of the year, 1981. Note the higher, more animated stride of the dressage horse. Note also the engagement of the hind limbs. *(Photograph by Terri Miller)*

a higher outside rim, because they run mostly on dirt or sand rather than turf. Thoroughbred racehorses wear light-weight aluminum shoes with large steel toe grabs. The lightness of their shoes allows them maximum striding and less fatigue on their legs. The steel toe grabs dig into the track surface so the horses can carry themselves far with each stride. Specially designed shoes are used for mud or turf. These shoes can affect the outcome of a race, so much that their use is posted on the equipment or tote board if they are being used.

Standardbred racehorses, trotters, and pacers are shod very differently. Because of the nature of their gaits, the narrowness of their sulky shafts, and the speeds they travel, their shoeing is probably the most diverse and difficult to master. The names of their shoes are as exotic as the racing game itself. Half-round, full swedge, half swedge, crossfire, Canadian bar, and mushroom bar are just a few types of shoes used on Standardbreds. Each one has a purpose, either to hold or not hold the track's surface. The lengths of the horse's feet and the angles are so precise that they are measured in sixteenths of an inch and are shod as often as ten days apart.

Jumpers, especially in the higher open and Grand Prix divisions, also need traction. Rim shoes would not provide sufficient traction, so calks or heels are used instead. Sometimes these are left in the shoes. At other times, holes are drilled and tapped into them so the calks can be removed or changed according to ground conditions. Eventers also make use of these removable studs, since they go from a level dressage area to the grueling, unpredictable cross-country course, then back into an arena to jump the stadium round during the course of a competition. If rain falls during this time, conditions can change. It would be impractical to reshoe the horses, so the studs are removed, added, or exchanged.

Dressage horses and show hunters are the ballerinas of the show world, and their gaits must show a long, elegant, and forward stride. In both cases, this long, low stride is encouraged; however, the higher the level the dressage horse attains, the more his center of balance moves to the rear. As this happens, the dressage horse frees his shoulders more and moves in higher

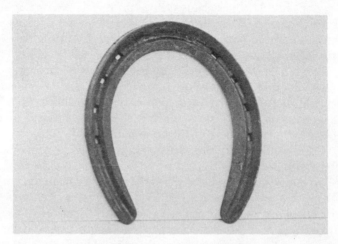

Barrel racing shoe. Note the high, outside rim for traction.

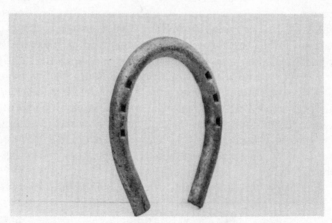

Half-round front shoe with unfinished heels.

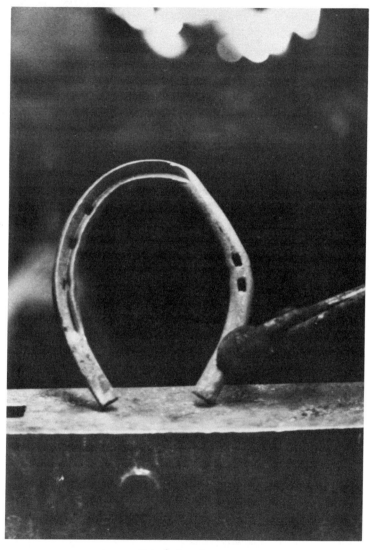

A crossfiring shoe for a pacer.

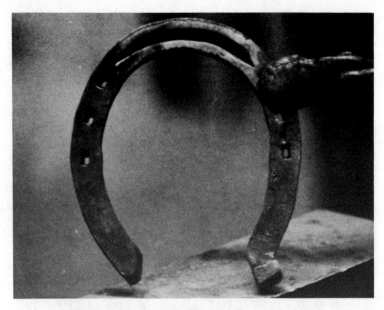

Hind shoe with trailer, block heel, and creased toe.

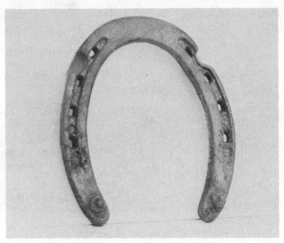

Hind keg shoe with drive-in calks.

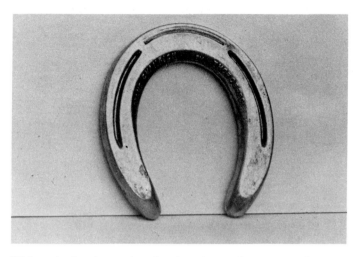

Wide-web aluminum shoe for show horse, dressage, or hunter.

action, but still has long strides as opposed to the higher, shorter stride of the Saddlebred horse.

Aluminum shoes are used quite often on dressage horses and hunters, but they are of a much different type. The aluminum shoes they wear are thicker than their racing counterparts. The steel toe grab is replaced by a steel plate so the softer aluminum won't wear too quickly. Removable calks are sometimes used on higher-level dressage horses so that they can perform pirouettes and flying changes every stride on less than ideal footing.

Show hunters are judged on conformation and way of going and on the way they move in the hack classes. The judges like to see a horse move long and low, what they call "daisy cutting," moving freely from the shoulder. Because their balance is more on the forehand, they travel lower than the dressage horses. Their jumping rounds must be smooth and fluid. Shoeing can't help a horse use his knees better; however, a comfortable horse in balance will perform his best.

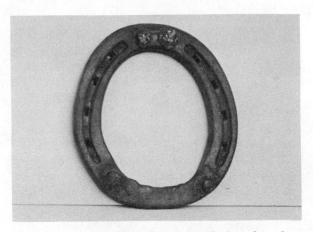

Egg-bar shoe with borium studs, made from keg shoe.

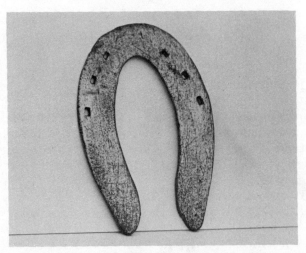

Hind reining plate for longer slide stops. Extreme width provides low friction to allow the longer slide.

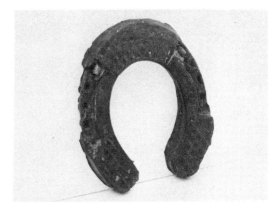

Rubber horseshoe used by some police horses, street carriage horses, and some types of circus horses.

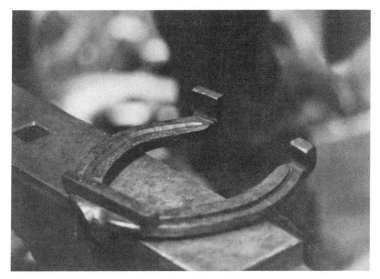

A well-made draft-horse shoe made by Edward Martin of Scotland.

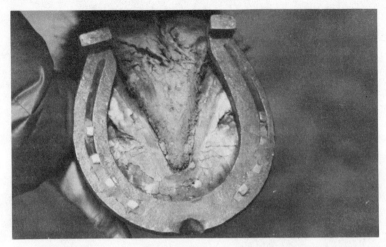

Properly made and fitted hind-draft horseshoe by Edward Martin.

Field hunters and endurance horses move quickly over varying terrain and cover a great deal of ground. Beauty of movement is not as important as function in this case. More durable types of shoes are used on these horses, usually with the carbide alloy borium welded to the shoes. This borium is very hard and comes in different grits to allow more or less traction or wear.

Traction is absolutely nonexistent in reining horses. Their hind shoes are very wide (at least ⅞ inch to 1¼ inches wide), and the nails used are filed down flush so that the horses can literally sit on their hocks and slide great distances.

Now that you understand why horses need special shoes, let's see how they work. Swedges, or rims, fill with dirt and act as sandpaper to be abrasive to the ground. Weight can add action either for height or reach, depending upon where it is placed. Weight can also alter foot flight to prevent interference. Lightness in shoes aids in natural movement and eases fatigue. Shoes that do not hold the horse back are half-round and flat, wide-web shoes. A wide-web shoe, whether aluminum or steel, takes weight bearing off the wall and distributes it better over a larger portion of the foot.

7

Caring for Unshod Feet

Some horses do not require shoes. It is an old saying that shoes are a necessary evil. If applied correctly, shoes are an asset and are especially useful for traction and protection. Four to eight weeks is the approximate time span for the feet to grow between shoeings. Over the winter, the feet usually grow a little slower and riding time is limited, so six weeks can run into eight weeks between shoeings, but resetting is always necessary.

Most young horses only get front shoes during their training to avoid accidents to their limbs. Some people believe they should remove the shoes for a couple of months a year to let the feet grow. Properly fitted shoes will not harm the feet in any way; however, if the shoes are left on all winter with no resets or trimming, it can be very detrimental to the hooves. If you do decide to pull the shoes, regular trimming is still necessary to maintain strong, healthy feet throughout the shoeless period. If the feet are not cared for during this time with regular trimming, the farrier may have a difficult time reshoeing the horses when that time comes. Much of the time, feet will not grow out perfectly straight due to conformation, etc. Feet left all winter untrimmed and unbalanced will be stubby and difficult to bring back into condition, requiring several months to grow out properly again. It is a good idea for broodmares to have their shoes removed before foaling time to avoid causing injury to the foal. Foals should have their feet handled soon after birth. Trimming

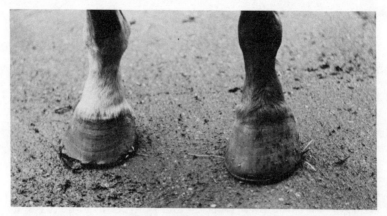

Feet in need of new shoes.

is not usually necessary for six to twelve weeks. The hoof is too soft to trim for the first four weeks; after that, periodic trimming is necessary. A bit of "toeing out" is normal for young, leggy foals because of the way they must stand to reach the ground while grazing. If excessive toeing out is noticed, or toeing in, or any other limb deviation, it should be cared for accordingly. Correction should be started early and continued regularly for best results. Feet should be cleaned daily, whether shod or barefoot. When necessary, hoof dressing should be applied so that the feet remain pliable and healthy. The heel of the foot, as well as the frog, should be flexible, so that every time the horse steps down on his feet it will expand and contract with pressure. This is the normal movement of the foot.

When trimming the foot to leave it bare, it should be trimmed exactly the same as if a shoe were going to be put on. This means it should be balanced properly and trimmed correctly. You may want to leave a little more sole than normal, because the sole is the natural protection for the foot against

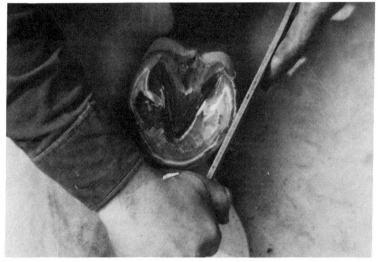

Rounding off the wall of the hoof of a foal or barefoot horse to prevent splitting of the wall. *(Photograph by Anthony Cordero)*

rocks and bruises. The wall should be trimmed a little higher than the sole and then beveled at a 45-degree angle to prevent chipping. If chips do occur between trimmings, the horse owner can take a file or rasp and gently rasp them off so they will not tear. If the horse's feet persist in cracking and splitting badly, the farrier should be called and the shoes replaced.

8

Common Problems

Our horses are plagued by many problems that can be aided by prudent, corrective shoeing and trimming. Many of these problems occur through changes in use, old age, and arthritic conditions such as spavin, sidebones, and ringbone. These are all inflammations of cartilage surrounding joints. In the bulk of these cases, once the inflammation ceases its growing or active stage (manufacturing and setting of calcium) the pain will subside. During the recuperative period, which may take months, it is sometimes very painful for the horse to move the affected joints. The goal of corrective shoeing here is to minimize movement by trimming and by using a helpful half-round shoe. Pads will help absorb shock, and degree pads provide aid in reducing movement. In the case of spavins in the hock, a shoe with a long trailer and a rolled toe helps breakover and stabilizes the hock joint. Trimming the toes shorter and raising the hoof angle helps.

Navicular problems usually develop in certain conformation types. If a horse has small feet and short, stumpy pasterns, much shock is absorbed in the bone. Over a period of time, the bone will start to develop small spurs which irritate the deep flexor tendon as it travels over its pulley, the navicular bone. The calcium itself does not hurt the horse, rather it is this action over the tendons which hurts. There are many nerve endings in this area which make it very sensitive to pain. Bar shoes are very helpful, as are degree pads with foam rubber or silicone packing to protect the heel area. Rolling the toes or using half-

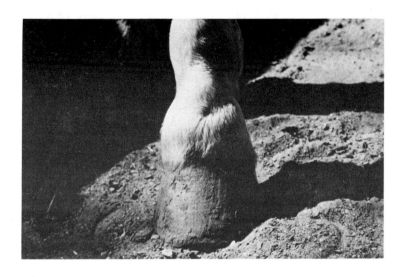

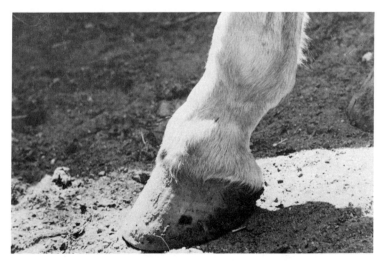

Ringbone on left front foot. Notice enlargement above coronet band.

round shoes minimize navicular problems as well. Sheared heels indicate a condition whereby the soft tissue which holds the heels together over the frog is torn by unequal pressure or overreaching. This is sometimes mistaken for navicular problems, because the horse will favor the same area and limp similarly. Wide-web bar shoes, either egg bar or regular bar shoes, depending on conformation, will be used to hold the heels together so that they can heal. The most important correction is the proper trimming of the feet to equalize the pressure on the heels.

Most people don't realize it, but horses are subject to bruises or corns. Bruises can result from a blow from a hard object, such as a rock or hard ground, and corns are caused by improperly fitted shoes. Sometimes a well-fitted shoe is left on too long, and as the foot grows and spreads out, the shoe does not spread with it. When this happens, it may rest on the buttress where the heel and white line meet to fit into the bar. This area is easily bruised, and when a corn develops or a bruise occurs, a pad made of leather or plastic should be applied with either hoof packing or silicone to protect the area. Bruises or corns left unattended can turn into abscesses, where the capillaries fill with blood and put tremendous pressure on the area. Abscesses should be drained, either by soaking till they break or by cutting them open and allowing them to drain before a shoe is applied. The cutting out of abscesses should be done by a veterinarian, because antibiotics may be needed, depending upon the depth, amount, and severity of the infection.

Sometimes even the best farriers make mistakes, and a nail can be driven improperly. In some cases, the area we have to work on is only $1/16$ of an inch or less. A close nail occurs when the shaft of the nail in its driven path through the wall bulges it slightly. This may, in cases of very thin walls, put pressure on the sensitive laminae, causing lameness. If the nail is removed quickly, the lameness should disappear. Sometimes soaking in Epsom salts or poulticing the horse's foot will ease inflammation. Iodine or betadine solution should be applied to the area as well.

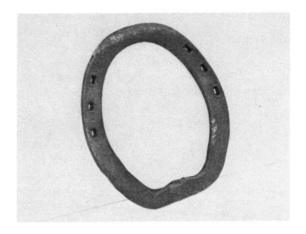

Quarter-by-¾ bar shoe suitable for navicular disease or sheared heels.

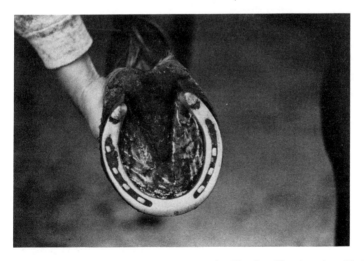

In need of new shoes. Notice overgrowth of heels, allowing the old shoe to rest on the buttress, causing corns.

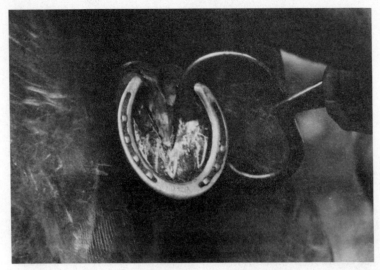

Using hoof testers to check the sole for bruises or soreness.

Sometimes the nail can go directly into the sensitive tissue, causing what is called a quick. The nail draws blood and causes a more serious condition which may develop into an infection or an abscess if left untreated. The derelict nail should be pulled immediately. Sometimes pouring iodine into the hole will be sufficient. In more severe cases, the shoe must be pulled and the foot poulticed. Any infection must be stopped with antibiotics.

Daily care of your horse's feet should include cleaning out with a hoof pick and checking for lodged stones, which can cause bruises. Notice the condition of the frog of the foot. It is an excellent indication of hoof texture. A quick squeeze should tell you if it is too dry. A healthy frog should have the consistency of a rubber pencil eraser. If it is too dry, a good commercial hoof preparation should be applied. Some of these are too thick and should be thinned out a bit by heating or mixing with vegetable oil. An excellent hoof dressing you can make is one part pine tar, one part vegetable oil, and one-half part Venus of Turpentine.

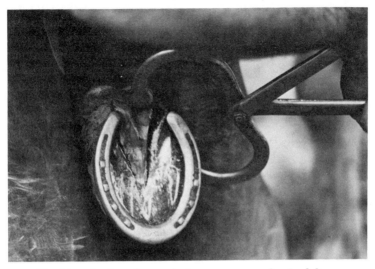

Checking the frog for navicular soreness or bruised frog.

Venus of Turpentine, used on the soles and heels of a horse's feet, aid in toughening and adding resilience to help prevent bruises. It should be left in the sun or heated to soften in order to achieve the maximum effect. If you find, while cleaning your horse's frog, that it is very soft, emanating a foul smell, and has a thick black substance around it, your horse probably has thrush. The best cure and prevention for thrush is a clean, dry stall. A buildup of the bacteria in urine and manure in the foot will rot the frog. Stalls and feet should be cleaned daily. If your horse does get thrush, have your farrier pare away as much diseased tissue as possible, then flush the area with some bleach and water in equal parts and apply a commercial thrush remedy. Care should be taken so that the bleach does not burn the tender skin above the foot.

Water and mud won't hurt your horse's feet. The capillary action in the wall will only absorb so much moisture. A much larger danger to the feet is the buildup of gooky hoof dressing.

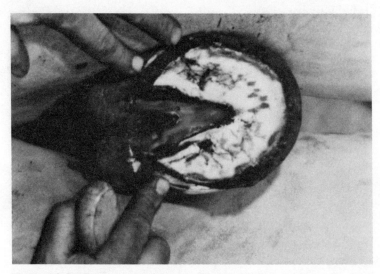

Hoof with badly contracted heels. *(Photograph by Anthony Cordero)*

Too much hoof dressing rots the wall under it until it will no longer hold nails. Ultimately, the hoof falls apart. The practice of painting a horse's feet before each class should be discouraged. There are hoof polishes on the market that keep the feet shining all day with just a damp rag and are better for the feet.

CRACKS

Small cracks in the wall of the hoof are usually not harmful to the horse, and their appearance is merely a cosmetic blemish. Cracks are a sign of brittle or dry feet and should be treated by soaking and applying a good hoof dressing to encourage the foot to become more pliable during growth. There are nutritional supplements that aid in this process by encouraging the hoof to grow at a faster rate. There are many products on the market that claim this ability. Horses are individuals, and what works on one may not work on another. Trial and error will determine what works best for your horse.

Larger cracks or quarter cracks can be very painful, as they are widened and opened by the horse's steps. The sensitive lamina inside may be pushed out through the crack. When the horse picks his foot up, it pinches this tissue between the sides of the fissure and causes extreme pain. The hoof should be stabilized by use of a wide-web bar shoe with clips, and the area directly under the crack should have about $1/16$ of an inch free space to take away all pressure. Enough room to slide in a hacksaw blade is sufficient to relieve pressure, yet it allows foreign material to enter and cause further problems. Application of Venice of Turpentine to the affected area of the hoof and crack encourages it to grow faster.

In severe cases, a crack may be stabilized by literally tying it shut with screws and wire. Small holes are drilled on either side of the crack through the wall. Either wire is used to actually sew it together, or a small metal plate is screwed in both sides over the crack. This is usually not necessary unless the crack is very deep and very large. It will sometimes take a year and a half for a crack to grow out, depending on its severity. The crack will remain in the hoof until the new hoof at the top of the coronet band reaches the ground. This is the normal length of time for the hoof to grow out completely, in most cases.

COMMON HOOF PROBLEMS

Problem

Correction

Abscess

Trim away or soak foot until abscess breaks and drains. When horse can walk soundly, shoe with pads and pack abscess cavity with cotton soaked in iodine.

Broken or worn-down walls
Apply rim pads or full pads to relieve pressure on the sole.

Contracted heels
Balance feet, achieve frog pressure. If possible, fit shoes full with beveled heels to encourage spreading. Using ¾ shoes or leaving the hoof barefoot is good. Keep hoof pliable.

Contracted tendons
Balance feet, using ¾ shoes or tips, and give the horse long, slow exercise daily.

Corns or stone bruises
Use wide-web shoes with pads, or wide-web aluminum shoes. Concave the shoe so that the shoe does not rest on the corn. Soak hoof till pain subsides.

Cracks (toe)
Use wide-web bar shoes with clips on either side of the crack to stabilize it. Cut or burn a groove across the top of the crack to retard further cracking.

Cracks (quarter)
Use wide-web bar shoes with clips on either side of the crack. Leave a small space under the crack to relieve pressure and/or lameness. Burn or cut a groove across the top of the crack.

Forging
Elevate front angles / speed breakover. Front shoes may have rolled toes, square toes, or can be made of ½ round steel. Hind shoes may have a square toe, heels, or trailer.

Founder or laminitis
Very wide-webbed shoes with concaved hoof surface take pressure from flat sole. Trim feet according to the new position of the coffin bone if it has rotated, and use thick, soft pads or double pads (stiff to ground, soft to sole) with silicone packing.

Interference
Lower the outside of front feet and use a square or rolled toe shoe. Lower the outsides of hind feet and use a trailer, square-toed shoe, crossfire shoe, or side weight.

Nail prick	Remove offending nail. Flush with iodine or peroxide if bleeding is present and soak foot if horse is lame.
Navicular disease	Use a wide-web or bar shoes, ½ round or aluminum shoes, with degree pads, silicone, or foam rubber packing. Roll or square toes of shoes, balance feet or slightly elevate angles if conformation warrants.
Padding/winging	Properly balance feet, adjust shoe weight, either lighter or heavier, roll or square toe.
Puncture wounds	Remove foreign object carefully if still embedded in hoof. Cleanse wound thoroughly. Soak foot until horse walks sound, then shoe as if for an abscess. Call vet immediately for antibiotics and tetanus booster.
Sheared heels	Balance foot's lateral axis properly and apply a wide-web bar shoe to relieve pressure, and treat the thrush which usually accompanies this.
Sidebone	Use wide-web shoes fitted full under the sidebone; use pads or ½ round shoes.
Stumbling	Elevate angles with a rolled or squared toe: also a ½ round shoe can be useful. In the case of a horse decidedly over at the knee, proper balance is very important. Do not raise angles too severely, as this will also cause stumbling, and the horse will rock over the toes too quickly and fall onto its knees.
Thrush	There is no particular shoeing to help this condition. Clean, dry stalls are the best prevention. If thrush does occur, trim away as much diseased tissue as you can from the frog and treat with a thrush remedy or flush with peroxide or bleach, then treat with iodine.
Toed out	Usually lower outside slightly.
Toed in	Usually lower inside slightly.

Feet trimmed too short or worn-down walls	Bevel hoof surface of a wide-webbed shoe or apply pads or rim pads to relieve pressure on the sole.
Weak walls	Use wide-web lightweight shoes, such as aluminum fitted with smallish nails well-driven. Start good nutritional program and use proper hoof preparations to strengthen walls.

9

Limb and Gait Deficiencies

If you looked at your horse's legs through an engineer's eyes, you would be surprised and amazed at how such fragile structures can function as marvelously as they do. The limb is made up of a series of bones, ligaments, tendons, soft connective tissue and hard tissue called horn. The joints will work very well for a number of years, trouble-free, if one does not interfere with their particular balance. When man tries to change the natural way an adult horse is built, unnatural strain is placed on the joints, tendons, ligaments and other structures.

One of the ways nature has allowed for mistakes to be dealt with in limb deviations ties in the hoof itself. A hoof will tell an experienced eye many things about what has happened in the recent past. It takes about a year for the hoof to grow from the coronary band to the ground surface. In this period, any injuries or stressful situations will show up as scars or rings in the hoof wall. Any deviation of balance will also become apparent, as one side of the hoof wall will flare out, while the other will grow straight or even turn inward and contract. Any pain in the higher part of the limb will show, because the lame leg will sometimes have a contracted foot due to the decreased amount of weight the horse will bear on it.

A healthy hoof will grow symmetrically and expand and contract rhythmically with each stride, disbursing any concussion away from the upper limb. Most limbs, unfortunately, are not of the ideal kind, so we and our horses must cope with what we have. Some horses stand squarely on their feet, but when they move, deviations occur. Others stand crooked, but move straight. These individuals are much better off than their prettier counterparts. A horse with a deviation in stance, followed by a straight gait, is much more likely to be sound and remain that way. Certain problems can be dealt with through corrective trimming or shoeing till about the age of fourteen months, when the foal has reached about 80 percent of his adult height. After this period, the growth plates at the end of the bones of the joints have become hardened, and further correction can be dangerous.

In severe cases or in cases of expensive stock, an operation called stapling can be performed, whereby the longer or faster growing side of a joint can be fastened together, allowing the shorter side a chance to catch up. After a period of time, the staples are removed and the joint will grow straight. Careful evaluation of a prospective purchase should be made, including his feet in stance and his way of going. Don't buy a poor prospect at a cheap price and expect your blacksmith to perform miracles.

In adult horses, the degree of correction should be only to get the feet back into proper balance for that individual, whether it is aesthetically pleasing or not. As long as the gait deviation does not cause interference or undue strain on the limb, the saying, "What you see is what you get" applies.

In some cases, the limbs are straight, but the hooves themselves don't match each other. One foot may be a little more upright than its mate, or one a little larger or rounder. These are usually due to differences in the bone structure of that particular limb. Perhaps the pastern of one leg is a bit shorter or the shape of the coffin bone is different. The feet should be trimmed to match their respective limbs, regardless of appearance. This is the way that the horse is made, and common sense should always prevail as to trimming and shoeing. The following are some examples of common limb and hoof deviations and deficiencies. Again, common sense and an understanding of the mechanics of how the joints, tendons, etc., interact must be your guide.

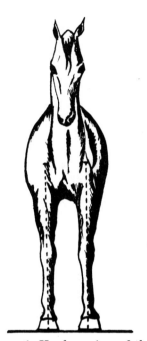 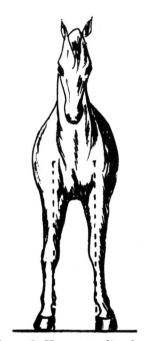

Figure 1. Head-on view of the forelimbs of the horse in the normal position.

Figure 2. Horse standing base-wide. Note the position of the forelegs outside the vertical line.

Figure 1. This is the ideal horse, a leg in each corner squarely placed so that the horse will remain in balance no matter in which direction he is going. He will probably be very versatile and remain sound a long time.

Figure 2. This shows a horse standing base-wide with his toes pointed outward. This individual will probably have a rolling gait, and, because of the wideness of the limbs, will not interfere, but in extreme speed he could possibly cross his front legs and stumble. Most foals stand this way because their legs are too long for their necks. They usually outgrow this stage by approximately ten months of age, and it should not be of any major concern, as long as the foal travels straight. This happens

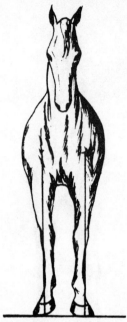 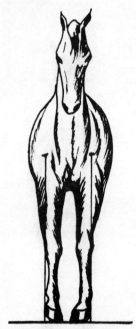

Figure 3. In the "toe-wide" position, the toes are pointing outward. As the animal moves forward, the pattern of flight of each foot takes the shape of an outward arc rather than the normal straight line in which the feet should travel.

Figure 4. In the "toe-narrow" or "pigeon-toed" position, the toes are pointing inward, and the pattern of flight of each foot takes the shape of an inward arc.

because foals must stand with their front legs spread apart to graze or to nurse; consequently, the inner wall of the hoof grows a bit straighter and the outside wall flares a bit. Monthly trimming should bring the hoof back into balance, but care should be taken not to overtrim to correct this.

Figure 3. This is the toe-wide position, and this animal has a harder time traveling because his limbs are set closer together. This horse will probably interfere, or worse, stumble quite often, because he swings his legs in an inward arc every stride.

Figure 4. The toed-in or pigeon-toed horse experiences fewer problems; because of the outward swing of flight, interfer-

Flight pattern of front feet
Normal   Toe-In   Toe-Out

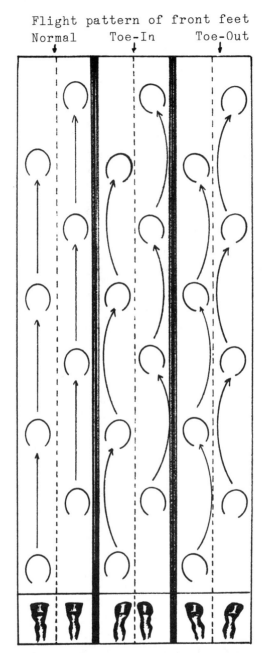

Figure 5. Flight pattern of front feet. Normal.
Toe-In. Toe-Out.

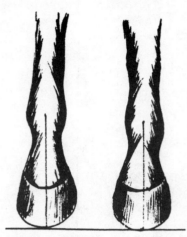

Figure 6. Closeup of front feet in the normal position.

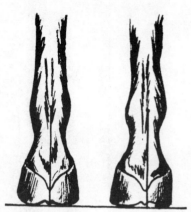

Figure 7. Closeup of front feet as seen from behind.

ence is less likely to occur. Horses with this conformation have an easier life than those who toe out. This puts less strain on the splint bones and joints of the ankle, making for a more useful horse.

Figure 5. This shows the flight patterns of the toed-out and toed-in hoof. Take notice that the inward arc of the toed-out horse crosses that imaginary line where interference can occur. Also notice that the longer or wider the arc, the longer that foot is in the air, causing more prolonged strain to its accompanying foot.

Figures 6 and *7* are closeups of normal feet as shown from the front and from behind. Note the symmetry and balance of these hooves and how the flexion of the hoof can be used to its fullest advantage to absorb shock.

Figures 8 and *9* show toe-wide or base-wide feet pointing outward. The difference in the length of the inside and outside walls is apparent, and correction would involve lowering the outside wall as close as possible to the T-square through the pastern as discussed in balancing the foot.

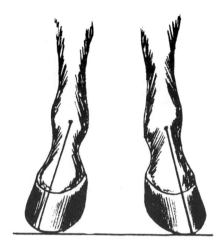

Figure 8. Closeup of "toe-wide" or base-wide front feet.

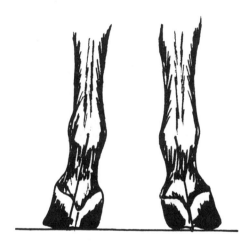

Figure 9. "Toe-wide" or base-wide feet as seen from behind. (Please note the change in the angle of the foot, which is outward.)

Figure 10 shows the toe-narrow or base-narrow feet again as seen from the front and from behind. This is the opposite problem. Notice that now the inside wall must be lowered to achieve correct lateral balance. Again, only enough correction should be done to achieve as close to the perfect T-square as possible without excessive twisting of the limb.

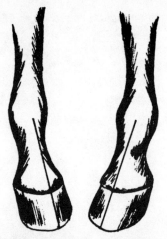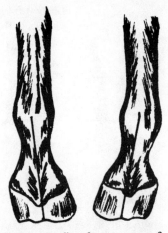

Figure 10. Closeup of "toe narrow" or base-narrow feet from the front. Please note hoof angle broken inward.

"Toe-narrow" or base-narrow feet as seen from behind.

The lateral balance is the deciding factor in the flight or forward movement of the limb. Mild gait or stance deviations in adult horses should be left alone if the balance is correct for that limb. The only time more severe measures should be taken is when interference or excessive twisting is noticed. If you have any doubts when purchasing a new prospect as to straightness or soundness, have a veterinarian or competent farrier recommend the best course to take and advise you if the problem can be solved or lived with. There are very few perfect horses, but a great many flight problems are caused by poor or neglectful hoof care. If a shoe is too heavy or the angle of the hoof is incorrect, climbing or excessive knee action could result. On the other side of the coin, feet out of balance laterally will create bizarre flight patterns, sometimes resulting in lameness.

Figures 11 and *12* show that the hind limbs of a horse can also have their share of problems. Figure 11 shows a base-narrow stance behind. Even in correctly conformed horses, the hind legs travel a little closer together; consequently, more interference occurs here. The basic principle of correction still applies: to make the foot laterally balanced again so weight is

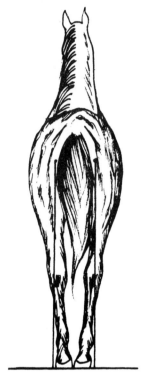 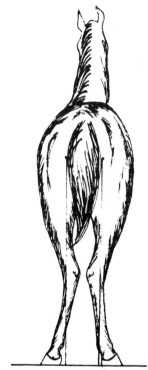

Figure 11. Base-narrow
stance as seen from behind.

Figure 12. "Cow-hocked" or
base-wide stance.

borne equally on both sides. In this case, lowering the inside
wall would be indicated. This may cause the feet to stand a little
toe-out; however, the gait will be more correct. Figure 12 shows
the cow-hocked horse with the opposite problem, the correction
of which is to lower the outside. Here again, we will alter stance
and gait, hopefully for the better. In correcting problems in the
hind feet, we have the advantage of using a shoe with a trailer
on it. These cannot be used in front for fear of the hind feet
catching them. The trailer can create a longer ground surface,
causing the affected limb to stay on the ground a bit longer and
allowing for the clearance of its mate.

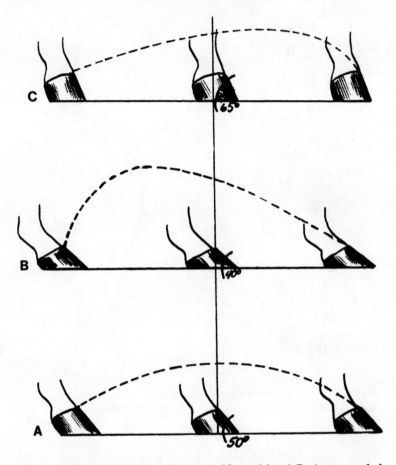

Figure 13. Side-view of hoof flight. *A*. Normal hoof. *B*. Acute-angled hoof. *C*. Upright hoof.

Figure 13. The medial balance of the hoof is the balance from the toe to the heel, making the alignment correct for the bones above. This measurement determines the height of the arc in flight.

Figure 14 shows the stance of the normal horse with correct medial balance.

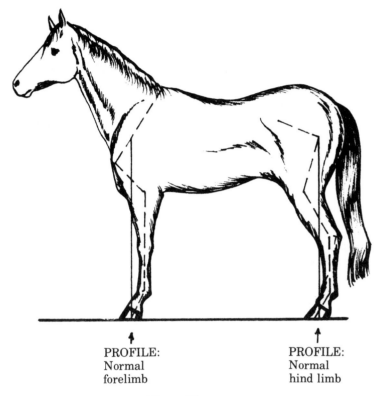

PROFILE:
Normal
forelimb

PROFILE:
Normal
hind limb

Figure 14.

Figure 15. Horses with these defects should have their toes shortened judiciously to try to get the hoof back under the mass. If too much trimming is attempted or the foot is built up too high with the use of degree pads, knuckling over or falling could occur. Worse yet would be the problem of tearing of the toe because of increased pressure.

Figure 16 shows the horse over at the knee and standing under. This horse should have the heels slightly lowered to help place the feet under the body better.

Ideally, a line dropped through the leg should fall directly behind the bulbs of the heels. This would allow the lever action of the joints above their maximum support.

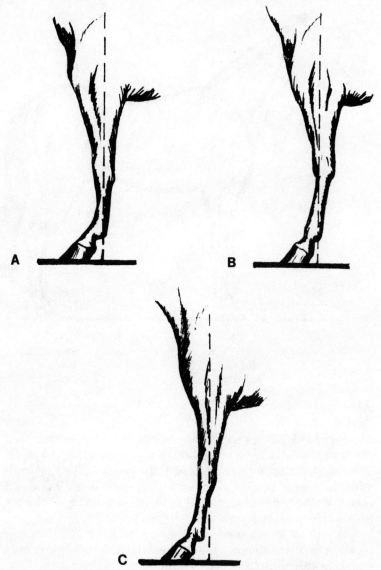

Figure 15. A. A low-jointed or acute-angled foot; *B.* "Calf-kneed" or "sheep-kneed"; *C.* Leg placed too far forward or "camped in front."

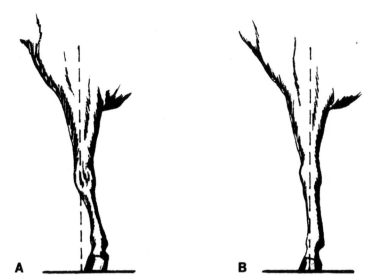

Figure 16.A. "Over in the knees" or knee-sprung; *B.* "Standing under" position.

In *Figure 17,* you can see how an upright foot is too far under the body, while an acute-angled hoof is too far forward, placing strain on the pasterns and tendons above. Corrective shoeing for these problems should be to fit the shoe very full at the toe of the upright hoof, thus slowing breakover without removing any toe when finishing off the hoof. The acute-angled hoof should have as much toe as can be removed safely, and in severe cases, the use of an egg-bar shoe is helpful to create the hoof that isn't there.

Figure 18 shows that the same thing can happen on the hind limbs. This horse has straight hocks and his feet "camped-out" behind the vertical line. Trim this horse's heels shorter to achieve better stance and gait.

Figure 19 demonstrates the opposite problem. This drawing shows that the hock is too angulated, creating a sickled or saber-hocked condition. Trimming the toes shorter and using a trailer is advised here to give the pastern more support. This

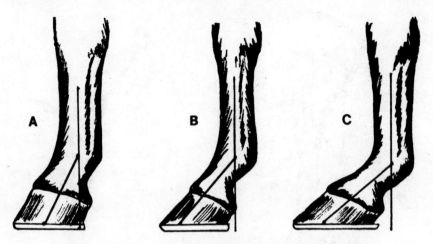

Figure 17. *A*. Upright; *B*. Normal angle; *C*. Acute-angled.

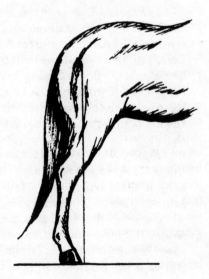

Figure 18. Side view of horse standing with hind legs "camped" behind the vertical.

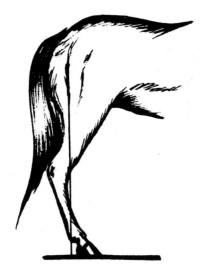

Figure 19. Side view of sickle-hocked, or "saber-legged" horse.

correction will slow the stride a bit to give the front legs a chance to gain clearance.

In *Figure 20,* the "bear" or "club foot" has its medial axis broken at the coronary band. Sometimes this is due to a slight rotation of the coffin bone or to faulty conformation in the pastern. Care must be taken to trim this foot's balance correctly in relation to itself and not to try to match it to the other three feet. This problem rarely causes lameness if the foot is balanced properly.

Figure 21 shows a "wry" foot which is not placed directly under the leg column. Most often, the foot is positioned to the outside. This causes a straight inside wall and a flared outside wall. The correction would be to balance as closely as possible to effect a correct distribution of weight and fit the shoe fully to the inside to try and compensate for the difference. A similar problem can be created if a farrier consistently trims one side of the foot lower than the other. Remember, the foot will always follow length, so the short side will get shorter while the longer side keeps flaring out.

Caution must be your byword in choosing, shoeing, or trimming your horses. A mistake made today might take a

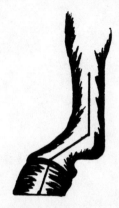

Figure 20. Bear or "club foot."

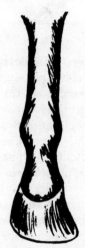

Figure 21. "Wry" or twisted foot.

couple of months or longer to show, but even longer to correct. The hoof grows constantly and slowly, and even while your farrier is working, every stroke of the rasp has its effect on what will happen six months from now.

10

The Farrier

When a farrier sets up an appointment to shoe a horse, it is his responsibility to arrive on time or let the horse owner know within a reasonable amount of time that he will be late. It is the horse owner's responsibility to be there when the farrier arrives or to return the courtesy of informing the farrier that it is necessary to make another appointment. The horse owner should have the horse inside in a dry, level area and, preferably, have the feet cleaned of manure and mud. There is nothing worse for a farrier's trimming tools than to have two inches of mud caked onto a horse's hooves. It ruins expensive nippers and even more expensive rasps. The mud cakes up into the rasp, and it is virtually useless afterwards.

Depending on where you live, certain times of the year can be better for shoeing horses. This does not mean that there is only one time you should call your farrier; rather, a few precautions can be taken to make the experience more comfortable for both horse and farrier. In hot weather, it is nice to have a cool, shady spot for the farrier to work in for two reasons: (1) It is physically more comfortable for the horse and the farrier, and (2) the coolness discourages flies, allowing the horse to stand more quietly for shoeing. There is nothing more frustrating than to try to hold a horse's leg up while the other three are being eaten by flies!

In inclement or cold weather, the horse should be shod in a dry, warm place. It is impossible to shoe horses tied to a fence in the snow, in mud, or on the side of a hill somewhere. A garage or any type of overhang is usually sufficient. If you are having your horse shod in your garage and it has an overhead door, the horse should not be held under this door. If the horse picks its head up and hits the door, the door has a tendency to rattle, scaring the horse. Make room in the back of the garage where the ceiling is higher, and plan to stay with the farrier until the job is completed. Do not ever tie horses to the runners or overhead doors. If the horse hits the door with its head and pulls back frightened, it can easily remove the runners and drag the door down around its legs and down your driveway.

Most farriers will be glad to answer questions while shoeing your horse. It is very useful to keep a note pad for your own use and helps avoid repetitious questions. Reading articles in magazines or books is very helpful to the horse owner's education. Keep in mind that the farrier deals with your horse as a unique individual, and his needs may differ from those of other horses, depending on his type and conformation, the work he does, and the area in which he lives. If you do have questions, by all means ask them, but remember that a competent farrier knows from experience what your horse will require. He appreciates your respect and trust. Prompt payment brings prompt service. The truth is, a farrier will sooner come to a customer with an emergency who pays his bills on time than to someone who owes him money. With today's economics, horses are a luxury, but we must always set aside enough for the necessities such as feed, shoeing, and veterinary care.

Emergencies will arise, but as far as shoeing goes, most professional farriers guarantee their work for about six weeks. If your horse throws a shoe within that period, the farrier will come and replace it at no charge, as long as he does not have to make a special trip, such as on a Saturday night before a show. In that case, a small service charge may be made. If the farrier does charge for a new shoe every time the horse loses one, and if the horse loses shoes consistently, it may be time to find another farrier. Prices for shoeing will vary somewhat from area to area, but most professional farriers will usually command a fair price for their work.

It may be difficult for those who shoe part-time, as a sideline, to properly care for your horse if he has a problem or needs corrective shoeing; he may not be available when you need him. Some of these shoers travel from place to place and are not always reliable, so it may be worth the extra dollar or two to have the local professional farrier work on your horse.

If the shoeing needs of your horse warrant the expertise of a certain type of farrier not available in your area, e.g., if you have a gaited horse, local farriers may not have experience with these shoeing methods. You must bring the horse to an experienced farrier, or the farrier must make an extra trip to you. In cases like this, the farrier may charge for the extra mileage to come do your horse.

11

Discipline and Restraint

Shoeing horses or simply working around them can be pleasant for horse and handler/farrier if the horse has been properly trained and has good manners. When a horse has good manners and has been properly disciplined, it leads quietly, does not balk, stands quietly on crossties or one tie, and stands for its handler while it is being worked upon. The well-mannered horse does not attempt to kick at or bite its handlers, nor does it constantly paw the ground where it is tied. It allows its feet to be picked up and worked upon without fidgeting. Occasionally, young horses, or horses which have never quite gotten the hang of balancing themselves on three legs while being shod, will have a tendency to lean on the farrier or handler. Horse owners can improve upon the horse's balancing abilities by working with their animals for short periods of time, picking up the feet carefully and praising or rewarding the horse when it makes the attempt to stand without leaning on its handler. Some horses have a bad habit of leaning badly on handlers or farriers, simply because they were not schooled or corrected for it to begin with. If a horse is a severe leaner, have someone hold the horse on a long shank. Another person then picks up the leg of the horse, and when the horse beings to lean in excess, stands away and releases the leg. The horse will soon learn that it cannot use the handler to lean upon, and the result will be a better-balanced horse. The horse will school itself to become more secure on three legs, as it does not like the element of surprise when its "leaning post" person is removed. The horse owner's schooling of his horse will be appreciated by the farrier, as he is working with sharp tools and nails, and accuracy is a must for a good shoeing job. Many unnecessary problems, cuts, and scrapes result from having to deal with an undisciplined horse.

It is important that the horse owner familiarize himself with certain methods of restraint for the safety of the horse and handler. A useful piece of equipment for restraint is the chain shank, which can be placed in many positions to gain leverage and control over the horse. A chain length of one foot to fourteen inches is sufficient. It should not be too long. The shank part, held in the hand, should preferably be of leather, because nylon could easily burn the handler's hand if the horse were to jerk quickly away. The most common method of restraint is to place the chain part of the lead shank over the horse's nose through the halter. It should be placed through the near or left side ring, over the halter, across the nose, and through the other side ring and then snapped to the center ring of the halter again. If it is snapped to the far side halter ring, when the chain is jerked, it will pull the halter into the horse's eyes. By snapping it to the center ring, it keeps the halter centered on the horse's head, giving the handler maximum leverage.

Another method is to place the chain under the upper lip of the horse. The chain should be placed through the near side ring, under the upper lip, against the gum, and then snapped to the other side ring. Steadily increasing pressure should never be applied; just enough pressure on the chain should be used to keep it securely in place. If the horse tries to kick or strike, a short jerk will usually regain the horse's behavior and attention. It puts pressure on the lip, as well as pressure on the sensitive area behind the horse's ears, where nerve endings are close to the surface. It has the same effect as a special bridle called a "war bridle." The war bridle may have a system of pulleys and ropes to maximize control. I have found, however, that a simple halter placed close behind the horse's ears, with the chain placed this way, is very effective in restraining uncooperative horses. Do not be alarmed if a little blood drips from the horse's gums. It is better to have this happen than to have the handler or farrier bleeding from an unruly horse. In essence, it is a small price to ensure safe control. Hopefully, this will

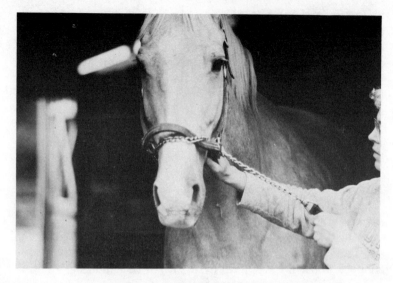

Proper application of nose chain.

serve as a training aid for the unruly horse and will not be needed in the future.

A twitch is sometimes used to restrain horses. A twitch can be homemade or purchased in a tack shop. It has a wooden handle about a foot to eighteen inches long with a six-inch loop of chain at the end. It is placed over the upper lip of the horse and tightened. Again, steady pressure should not be applied, just enough pressure to keep it in place so that if the horse reacts unfavorably, a tighter squeeze may be applied.

Sometimes twitches and war bridles only serve to make a horse more upset, especially nervous horses or horses who have had bad experiences with such things. Then it is time to call in a veterinarian or appropriate professional and administer a tranquilizer of some sort. This is a last resort and should be done carefully under the direction of the vet. It should never be attempted without the owner's permission, as some horses may have adverse reactions to tranquilizers or drugs of any kind. It is sometimes better to give a horse a mild tranquilizer and allow

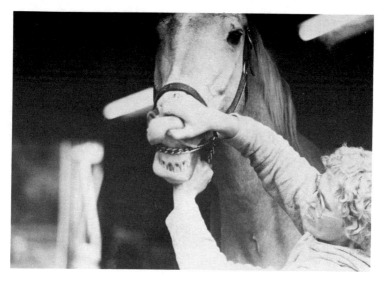

Application of lip chain to unruly horse.

him a good experience while being shod or handled so that subsequent trimmings or shoeings will be easier. Once he learns that the farrier or groom will not hurt him, he will accept such procedures more easily.

There are many methods of tying up a horse's legs, but I have found them to be dangerous for both the horse and the shoer and grooms, unless they are experienced in such procedures. If you do have to tie a horse up and put him on the ground to put shoes on, it should be done in a soft area to minimize the threat of injury. Throwing a horse or tying him up should be done only as a last resort, and the shoeing job done in this manner is not truly acceptable, because there is no way to check the balance when the horse is on its side, and you cannot sight the feet down correctly. It is much better to use other means to shoe the horse while standing than to throw him on his side. Training, "TLC," and good horsemanship will gradually make the horse more tractable.

Common sense should be used around horses at all times.

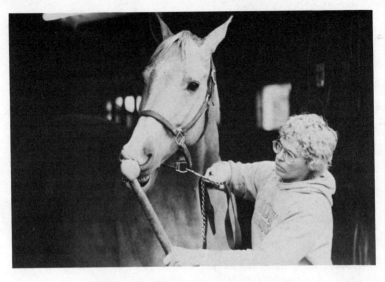

Application of twitch to undisciplined horse.

Sometimes the simple touching of a hot shoe to a horse's foot and the subsequent sizzling, or the little bit of smoke, is enough to send him tearing out of the barn halterless, leaving broken crossties or even broken bones in his path. In cold or bad weather, when the horse has been confined for a few days, the simple throwing down of a tool into a wood box may be enough to set him off. Observe the horse when he first comes out of the stall and see if he is calm or nervous. If the horse is nervous, care should be taken not to make matters worse. Work slowly and carefully around the horse and try to gain his confidence. If a horse appears calm, it is still advisable to work with caution, because the slightest thing can upset the best behaved horse. Crossties and halters should be made to give if a horse panics and tries to break away. One of the worst things that can happen is to have a horse fight a crosstie on a concrete floor with neither halter nor crosstie giving way. He can lose his footing, flip over backwards, and hang himself on the crossties. It is much better

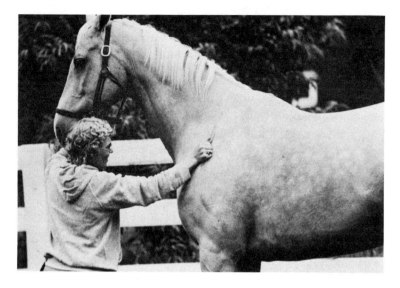

Pinching the nerves of the shoulder to restrain the horse.

to have at least one of the crossties break away and the other one hold, so that in case of an emergency, the horse will not hurt itself. If I am in a barn where the halters and crossties are very strong, I take a piece of baling twine, loop it through the halter, and attach the baling twine to the end of the crosstie. Should the horse panic, the twine will break, but the other crosstie will still hold the horse. This has saved many a horse and probably has saved me many a broken bone. Young horses, or horses that have not been handled very much, should never be crosstied and worked upon. Someone should always hold them. When working on foals for the first time, it is better to either go into the stall and have someone hold the mare with another person holding the foal next to the wall so that he can balance himself or to bring the two into a quiet, level area and again hold the foal where it can see its mother for reassurance. Pick up the foal's feet in a corner, so that it can balance itself against the walls. Remember, this procedure is acceptable for young foals, but as they grow and become accustomed to having their feet picked up, they should be discouraged from leaning on their handlers.

Try to work gently and cautiously, because the first few times you trim a foal will serve as his experience for subsequent shoeing and trimming. Poor handling of foals during trimming will only cause them to be afraid of the man with the apron, and the foal will have a lifetime of bad shoeing experiences ahead of him. The few extra minutes it takes when first trimming foals are certainly well worth it when they become yearlings and two-year-olds and need their first shoes. If foals have good experiences while being trimmed, their first shoes go on without a problem. It is often funny to watch them walk away with their first shoes on and see them stop and pick up their feet to see what this new sensation and noise is all about.

It is the horse owner's responsibility to spend enough time with his horses so that when the farrier arrives to shoe them, he is not working with a wild animal. If a horse is too hard to handle or is dangerous, a farrier should charge more or refuse to do such an animal without methods of restraint, tranquilization, or further training. A good farrier is a highly skilled professional who apreciates working on a disciplined horse.

12

Why Horses Lose Shoes

Your horse will sometimes lose, or "cast," a shoe, or it may become loose or shift on the foot. There are many reasons why this happens. The main culprit is mud. Deep clay mud will actually suck a shoe right off, clean as a whistle, without even damaging the wall. If this happens while you are out on the trail, try to walk home as uneventfully as possible, so as not to tear the wall of the hoof.

Shoes may also be tossed by being stepped on from behind. An excited horse turned out in a paddock will cavort airily, or set out to jump a six-foot fence and change its mind at the last moment, or set a new world's record for the slide stop into the fence. This will cause the hind feet to come up and catch the inside branches of the front shoes. A good pair of properly fitting bell boots will help prevent this while the horse is turned out. Never have the farrier shorten the front shoes, because this will cause corns and contracted heels. The hind shoes can have the toes slightly squared or rounded so as not to catch the front shoes so easily. Check the feet for proper balance so that the breakover speeds are correct. Adjustments must sometimes be made to either speed up the front or retard the hind feet. The use of a trailer or heels can help too.

Nails can sometimes break in the feet, causing the shoe to become loose. This usually happens to horses that travel with much concussion over hard surfaces. It is fairly common in trotters and pacers on hard winter racetracks. Riding horses usually don't suffer with this problem, except for some heavy jumpers who break nails in the front shoes.

During the hot, dry summer months, hooves go through many changes. Dry, hard ground makes the feet brittle, and the horse is more likely to shed a shoe because the walls don't expand and contract normally. If the horse casts a shoe in the summer, the walls usually break up more readily than at other times of the year. The best remedy, of course, is to maintain a healthy, pliable hoof with the use of dressing and moisture.

Summer insects are a big problem for horses. Insects around their legs annoy horses, causing them to stomp their feet on dry ground for hours, breaking nails and/or shifting shoes backwards. Insect repellents help alleviate this problem to some degree, but care must be taken not to drench the animals with insecticide. Some horses have allergic reactions to repellents. During the hottest part of a summer day, it may be a good idea to bring the horse into a shaded stall, if possible. Your horse will be more comfortable, and the risk of loosening shoes will be reduced.

Some horses are kickers in their stalls and will loosen their hind shoes by striking the walls with their feet. This vice should be discouraged. Sometimes moving the horse to another stall will solve the problem. Consistent kickers need stronger medicine, that is, the use of kick chains. These are six- to eight-inch-long chains, fairly heavy, which are strapped to the pastern of the offending legs. Each time the horse kicks, the chain comes back and strikes the horse.

Shoes also can come loose if the nails holding them are too small for the holes in the shoe, or if the heads of the nails wear down. The foot must be trimmed level and the shoe fitted to rest on the wall perfectly. If there is any rocking, the shoe will work its way loose all too soon. The clinches on the nails must be formed neatly and turned over to make a secure hook so they will not pop up with time. If the nails are not set deeply enough in the holes of the shoes, they will come up and become loose when the horse travels. The nails when driven should come out about ½ to ⅝ of an inch above ground surface for most riding or

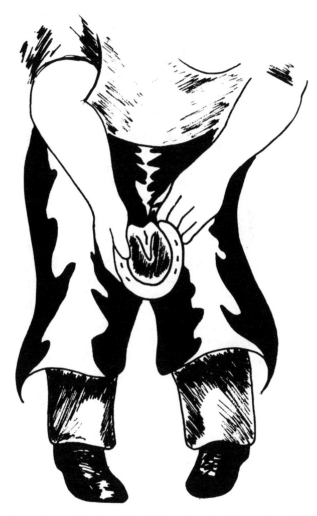

Correct positioning of the body when holding a front foot. Note that the toes point slightly inward for better support and balance.

racehorses. If enough time has lapsed since the last shoeing, the old holes should not present a problem in nailing. The line of the nails should be even, and no nails should be behind the bend of the quarters toward the heels. This practice would restrict the natural movement of the heels.

If your horse has a loose shoe, call your farrier. If the shoe is loose and twisted, there is danger of the hoof being penetrated by one of the other nails in the shoe. The shoe must be removed immediately. It is handy to have a shoe puller in your barn, especially if you have several horses. If you don't, a simple claw hammer and an old hoof rasp will do. Your farrier should be able to give you an old rasp. As I explained earlier, first file off the remaining clinches, then hold the foot and slide the claw of the hammer under the last remaining heel nail. Carefully pry the shoe upward and in toward the center of the foot. Care should be taken not to break the wall. As soon as the nail is loosened, tap the shoe back down to the foot. The nail should remain up. Pull the nail with the claw and carefully continue the process nail by nail until the shoe is off. Don't ride the horse on hard ground or turn him out until the farrier can replace the shoe. There is no need to remove the other shoe or shoes unless there is great discrepancy in angles if the horse is wearing degree pads. The best prevention for cast shoes is a regular schedule of farrier work, keeping the feet healthy with good nutrition, hoof preparations, exercise, and good grooming habits.

13

Coping with Emergencies

There are times in your horse's life when you, as a horse owner, will have to deal with various foot problems, such as a loose shoe, which should be removed, or a shoe that has been twisted or tossed. You should know what to do with the foot until the farrier arrives. If a shoe is loose (perhaps one or two nails are missing) but is still firmly on the foot, some electrical tape wrapped around the heels over the hoof will hold it on for a day or two until the problem is corrected. This is preferable to removing the shoe and possibly causing hoof damage. Sometimes a shoe is totally lost or is hanging on by one or two nails with some of the other nails protruding. In a case like this, the shoe should be removed immediately, as the protruding nails might enter, cut, or damage the foot. In order to do this, you should have a rasp and a pair of shoe pullers. If you don't have these tools available, any file will do to file down the remaining nail clinches on the horse's hoof; then a simple claw hammer placed directly under the nails still remaining in the hoof and gently pried toward the center of the hoof should allow you to remove the shoe safely. Never pry outward, as you may crack off part of the hoof. If the shoe is totally lost, you can gently level the edge of the wall to prevent any further chipping or cracking. In all cases, the farrier should be called immediately so that he can schedule your horse for a replacement of the shoe as soon as possible. The horse owner should not try to drive nails into the horse's hoof unless he has had previous experience. You can sometimes put a new nail into the old hole and gently turn over a clinch to help save the shoe, but caution should be taken in this procedure.

FIRST AID

First aid for your horse's feet may be necessitated by injury, disease, or accidents. There are certain things you can do to speed recovery until the veterinarian or farrier arrives. If your horse steps on a nail or a piece of glass or gets any type of a puncture in the foot, immediate lameness will be present in most cases. The object should be removed carefully, taking care not to leave any part of it in the foot. If possible, save the object causing the puncture for inspection by the vet or farrier. This will aid in determining if the entire piece has been removed. If the hole is not large enough to be seen easily, make a mental note of where it is so you can tell the vet. After removing the foreign object, clean out the wound with betadine, and scrub and soak the horse's foot in hot water to aid in removing any other foreign material that may have gotten into the hole (wound). Take some iodine ointment or antibiotic cream, apply it to the puncture, and cover the foot with a bandage. Place the horse in a clean, dry stall and call the vet. Tetanus vaccine (or booster) should be given to the horse upon the vet's arrival, because the tetanus toxoid lives and breathes in horse manure and in stalls, so any cut or puncture in the foot is very susceptible.

If, after riding your horse on hard ground, he appears foot-sore, he may have bruised the foot or the frog. If taking the horse into a soft area seems to make him more comfortable, chances are he has a bruise. The shoes do not necessarily have to be removed, but the vet or farrier should be called to try to localize the painful area by use of hoof tester or nerve blocking. If the bruise is in the foot, the foot should be soaked in hot water and Epsom salts. Following that, Venice of Turpentine should be painted over the sole and area of the bruise. After tenderness seems to leave the hoof, the next step is to reshoe the horse with pads. Pads will make the horse more comfortable when ridden until the bruise has a chance to grow out. In cases of very deep bruises or corns, an abscess sometimes develops, causing a pus pocket in the foot. Severe lameness will be noticed, and the pressure should be relieved by carefully trimming away the sole and allowing the abscess to drain.

In summer months, when the hooves get dry and the ground gets hard and sandy, horses with wide, flared feet may experience what is called separations in the quarters of the feet, especially the front feet. This occurs when the wall flares away from the white line and causes a small space where foreign material, such as sand, can work its way in. This becomes the separation itself. If the sand moves up high enough between the wall and the white line, it will cause pressure on the sensitive lamina and cause the horse discomfort and sometimes lameness. The shoes should be removed and the separation cleaned out with soaking of the foot to try to remove any residual material. The horse should be reshod with a wide-web shoe with quarter clips to keep the movement of the wall (especially at the heel area) to a minimum. Sometimes a bar shoe is called for, depending upon the size of the frog and the amount of movement. A pad with silicone packing should be applied, and cotton soaked with betadine or iodine should be placed into the separation. If this is taken care of properly, it should grow out as the foot grows, and wall and white line should come together again. Horses that are prone to separations should be shod a little more often, so that the heels do not spread out too far, with quarter clips kept on the shoes to minimize movement.

Separations can sometimes drag out for a long time and be very painful for the horse, and patience and good shoeing practices are the best cures or prevention. If the shoes are left on too long, another problem may arise. This is the problem of corns. Horses can get corns, just like people, from ill-fitting shoes. If the shoe is not fitted properly at the heel, as the hoof grows and spreads out, the shoe will put pressure on the sensitive portion of the sole at the heel area where the bar and the white line come together. This area is called the seat of the corn. Corns should be treated like bruises, and the hoof soaked and resuppled. Shoe the horse with a wide-web shoe and pad to protect the area until the corn grows out. Needless to say, the horse should be shod on a regular basis, with properly fitting shoes of the right type to support him in the best way possible.

14

Horseshoeing as a Career

In the United States, there are several associations or unions for farriers. Farriers who shoe horses at racetracks are members of the Union of Journeymen Horseshoers. They use the term journeymen because that is the way it is set up in their charter. You must be a member of the Journeymen association first, then apply for membership in the elite Union of Master Farriers or Master Horseshoers. There is also the American Farriers Association, which promotes good horseshoeing and educational services around the country and to which any interested person may apply for membership. Its headquarters are in Albuquerque, New Mexico, and Walter Taylor is the current President.

Opportunities in horseshoeing are unlimited. The horse industry is the fastest-growing part of the livestock industry today. The rapid growth of pleasure horse numbers, horse clubs, equestrian sports, horse shows, businesses related to the horse industry, and equine research make the future of horseshoeing look very good. Perhaps one of the most optimistic and attractive features about the horseshoeing business is the fact that horses' feet grow and change constantly and have to be cared for every four to six weeks. By 1980 the horse population in the United States, mostly pleasure horses, was reported to reach over nine million, and the horse industry has become a 17-billion-dollar-a-year business. Estimates are that more than fifty million people in the United States now ride or own horses, take lessons, or participate in equestrian sports.

Horseshoers who are highly skilled and competent are always in demand. In some areas, poor mechanics can get by and satisfy much of their public. It has been stated that about thirty percent of today's horse owners shoe their own horses. However, once horse owners are exposed to an expert, they can recognize the difference and will rarely go back to a less skilled horseshoer or continue to do their own horseshoeing. A man with his knowledge in his hands as well as in his head is invaluable.

Horseshoeing is an art and a skill, but it is also a science. Horseshoers must often work closely with veterinarians in treating conditions of the legs and feet of horses. A background in the sciences, and particularly in anatomy and physiology, is necessary when diagnosing, treating, and discussing ailments with a professional man such as a veterinarian. For this reason, and because a horseshoer is often considered to be an expert on horses, many are finding it advantageous to have some formal training at a college or university. The public should have as much confidence in their horseshoers as they do in their veterinarians. It takes time, study, and practice to become a skilled and proficient horseshoer.

Horseshoeing holds a great future for those who like to work and are willing to become skilled at it. There will always be room for a good horseshoer who is competent and dependable. If you choose to enter the profession, decide to become this kind of horseshoer; otherwise it is not worth the time and investment. There are few "naturals" in this business. A good craftsman is one who has knowledge in his hands. Practice makes perfect, especially in the horseshoeing business.

A good teacher is very valuable in studying horseshoeing, as in learning any trade. Good teachers are not always available and are not always the most popular, but they are the most effective. Evaluate your teachers carefully. Do they understand all they profess to know? Do they believe in what they teach? Are they constantly learning new things about the trade and improving themselves? Are they open to new ideas and innovations? These questions and others are important, because any teacher teaches what he is. Someone said that to be a horseshoer, one must have the strength of Sampson, the patience of Job, and the wisdom of Solomon. Others say all that is necessary is a strong back and a weak mind. You, the customer, must decide which of the two you wish to employ.

The practice of horseshoeing spans many fields. A horseshoer needs to be a horseman, blacksmith, businessman, and outdoorsman. The horseshoer must also be able to weld. It is helpful to understand how horses are trained and to have a thorough understanding of the structure of the horse's foot in order to work effectively with veterinarians.

Another trait that must be present or developed is the desire to work, and to work hard. There is no way to get around it. Horseshoeing is hard work. Piece work is also involved. When you don't work, you don't get paid, so, as you can see, a great deal of dedication is important in the farrier.

In the United Kingdom, there is a nationwide certification program that I feel should be adopted, in part, in the United States. As it stands now, any person who would like to become a farrier in this country needs only to purchase the tools of the trade and go out to unknowing clients. Luckily, the horse-owning public is becoming more aware of good shoeing practices and increasingly less tolerant of incompetence.

At the 1982 American Farriers Association Convention, I had the pleasure of talking with Edward Martin of Scotland, who is the President of the Master Farriers Association in the United Kingdom. He outlined for me how an apprentice farrier goes about getting into the trade. He must first apply to the agriculture department and get onto their waiting list. As openings for apprentices occur, they are moved up the list until a position is available. They then go to work for a master farrier for three years. During this time, they must also attend university courses in anatomy and physiology. After the three years, the apprentice must prepare for the nationwide board of examinations and pass them before he can work on his own as a journeyman. After another five years, application for the masters' association can be made, but only after competency has been proven.

Several states here have testing or certification, but there is

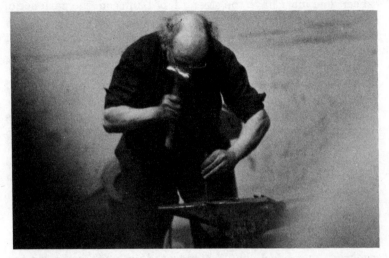

Edward Martin, President of the Master Farriers of the United Kingdom, at the American Farriers Convention, 1982.

no nationwide acceptance of this idea as yet. The American Farriers Association would like to see the certification of farriers in the United States. Shoeing horses is a very important and difficult job, and if a barber must be state-certified, I believe a farrier should be as well.

If you decide you want to become a farrier, there are many schools around the country. The length of the terms varies considerably, from two weeks to two years. A comprehensive list of schools can be obtained from state vocational boards or the Veterans' Administration. The American Farriers Association in Albuquerque, New Mexico, also has a list of schools that they consider to meet the requirements of the trade. Practice is the best teacher, and if you can find a competent farrier in your area who can take you with him, this experience would be very valuable for the apprentice or novice. Being a farrier carries a great deal of responsibility and should not be taken lightly. The rewards are few and the days long and hard, but I would not trade my life for any other.

Index

Feet, horse's (*cont.*)
 corns on, 74, 115–116
 first aid for, 114–116
 structure of hoof, 45–53
 trimming, 5–6, 22, 52, 54, 55,
  72
 See also Hoof
Fetlock, 35, 39, 41–42
Field hunters, 68
First aid, horse's feet, 114–116
Forging, 80
Founder, 80
Foundered foot, 56
Foundering horse, 22
Frog, 6, 45–46, 50, 51, 53, 56, 77
Fullered shoe, 10, 17
Full swedge, 61

Gait deficiencies, 83–85, 90–91
"Gravel," 23
Greek hippo sandal, 27

Half-round shoe, 61, 72
Half swedge, 61
Heels, contracted, 80
Hand-foot balance, 55
Hittites, 27
Hock joint, 41
Hoof, 35, 45–53, 78, 83, 84, 86,
  88, 92, 98, 110, 113–114, 115
 common problems with, 79–82
 cracks in, 78–79
 See also Feet, horse's
Horny sole, 50
Horses
 anatomy and physiology of
  legs, 35–44
 balance of foot, 54–58
 caring for unshod, 69–71
 disciplining and restraining
  while shoeing, 102–108

Horses (*cont.*)
 hoof structure, 45–53
 limb and gait deficiencies,
  83–98
 shoeing, 1, 5–10, 16, 18, 21–25,
  26–34, 52–53, 56, 72, 95, 97,
  99–101, 115, 117–121
 Shoes, 1–10, 10–17, 18–20,
  21–25, 30–34, 52, 59–68, 72,
  74, 79, 80, 81, 82, 109–110,
  112, 113, 115
Horseshoeing
 as a career, 117–121
 history of, 26–34
 See also Shoeing horses
Horseshoes, 72, 79, 80, 81, 82,
  115
 choosing shoes, 18–20
 history of, 30–34
 lameness, 21–25, 74
 loss of, 109–110, 112, 113
 need for shoes, 1–10, 52
 traction, 10–17
 types of, 59–68

Ice nails, 17
Inflation, effects of on shoeing
  horses, 32–34
Interference, 80
Internal foot, 48–51

Joints, 38, 41–43
Jumpers, 61

Knee spavin, 41

Lameness, 21–25, 56, 74, 90, 114
Laminae, 48
Laminitis, 18, 22, 80
Lateral, 35
Lateral balance, 55, 90